Advances and Trends in Clinical Microbiology: The Next 20 Years

Editor

JAMES E. KIRBY

CLINICS IN LABORATORY MEDICINE

www.labmed.theclinics.com

Editor-in-Chief
MILENKO JOVAN TANASIJEVIC

September 2019 • Volume 39 • Number 3

ELSEVIER

1600 John F. Kennedy Boulevard • Suite 1800 • Philadelphia, Pennsylvania, 19103-2899

http://www.theclinics.com

CLINICS IN LABORATORY MEDICINE Volume 39, Number 3
September 2019 ISSN 0272-2712, ISBN-13: 978-0-323-68223-7

Editor: Stacy Eastman
Developmental Editor: Laura Fisher

Reprints. For copies of 100 or more, of articles in this publication, please contact the Commercial Reprints Department, Elsevier Inc., 360 Park Avenue South, New York, New York 10010-1710. Tel. 212-633-3874, Fax: 212-633-3820, E-mail: reprints@elsevier.com.

Clinics in Laboratory Medicine (ISSN 0272-2712) is published quarterly by Elsevier Inc., 360 Park Avenue South, New York, NY 10010-1710. Months of issue are March, June, September, and December. Business and Editorial offices: 1600 John F. Kennedy Blvd., Suite 1800, Philadelphia, PA 19103-2899. Periodicals postage paid at NewYork, NY and additional mailing offices. Subscription prices are $274.00 per year (US individuals), $541.00 per year (US institutions), $100.00 per year (US students), $349.00 per year (Canadian individuals), $657.00 per year (Canadian institutions), $185.00 per year (Canadian students), $404.00 per year (international individuals), $657.00 per year (international institutions), $185.00 (international students). Foreign air speed delivery is included in all Clinics subscription prices. All prices are subject to change without notice. POSTMASTER: Send address changes to *Clinics in Laboratory Medicine*, Elsevier Health Sciences Division, Subscription Customer Service, 3251 Riverport Lane, Maryland Heights, MO 63043. **Customer Service: 1-800-654-2452 (US). From outside of the US and Canada, call 1-314-447-8871. Fax: 1-314-447-8029. E-mail: journalscustomerservice-usa@elsevier.com (for print support) or journalsonlinesupport-usa@elsevier.com (for online support).**

Clinics in Laboratory Medicine is covered in *EMBASE/Exerpta Medica, MEDLINE/PubMed (Index Medicus), Cinahl, Current Contents/Clinical Medicine, BIOSIS and ISI/BIOMED.*

Contributors

EDITOR-IN-CHIEF

MILENKO JOVAN TANASIJEVIC, MD, MBA
Vice Chair for Clinical Pathology and Quality, Department of Pathology, Director of Clinical Laboratories, Brigham and Women's Hospital, Dana-Farber Cancer Institute, Associate Professor of Pathology, Harvard Medical School, Boston, Massachusetts

EDITOR

JAMES E. KIRBY, MD, D(ABMM)
Associate Professor of Pathology, Harvard Medical School, Medical Director, Clinical Microbiology, Department of Pathology, Beth Israel Deaconess Medical Center, Boston, Massachusetts

AUTHORS

HENRIETTA ABODAKPI, PharmD, PhD
Department of Pharmacological and Pharmaceutical Sciences, University of Houston College of Pharmacy, Houston, Texas

JENNIFER DIEN BARD, PhD, D(ABMM)
Director, Microbiology and Virology Laboratories, Department of Pathology and Laboratory Medicine, Children's Hospital Los Angeles, Associate Professor of Pathology, University of Southern California, Los Angeles, California

ELLEN JO BARON, PhD
Cofounder and Board Member of Diagnostic Microbiology Development Program, Professor Emerita, Stanford University School of Medicine, Los Altos, California

THEA BRENNAN-KROHN, MD, D(ABMM)
Department of Pathology, Beth Israel Deaconess Medical Center, Division of Infectious Diseases, Boston Children's Hospital, Harvard Medical School, Boston, Massachusetts

ALEXANDRA L. BRYSON, PhD
Department of Pathology, Virginia Commonwealth University Health System, Richmond, Virginia

SHELDON CAMPBELL, MD, PhD
Department of Laboratory Medicine, VA Connecticut Health Care, Yale School of Medicine, New Haven, Connecticut

MARC ROGER COUTURIER, PhD, D(ABMM)
Medical Director, ARUP Laboratories, Associate Professor of Pathology, University of Utah, Salt Lake City, Utah

CHRISTOPHER D. DOERN, PhD
Department of Pathology, Virginia Commonwealth University Health System, Richmond, Virginia

THOMAS DURANT, MD
Department of Laboratory Medicine, Yale School of Medicine, New Haven, Connecticut

PETER H. GILLIGAN, PhD, D(ABMM)
Professor, Pathology-Laboratory Medicine, University of North Carolina at Chapel Hill School of Medicine, Chapel Hill, North Carolina

EMILY M. HILL, PhD
Pathology and Laboratory Medicine, Hunter Holmes McGuire VA Medical Center, Richmond, Virginia

JAMES E. KIRBY, MD, D(ABMM)
Associate Professor of Pathology, Harvard Medical School, Medical Director, Clinical Microbiology, Department of Pathology, Beth Israel Deaconess Medical Center, Boston, Massachusetts

ROSE A. LEE, MD, MSPH
Medical Microbiology Fellow, Department of Pathology, Beth Israel Deaconess Medical Center, Center for Life Science, Harvard Medical School, Fellow, Division of Infectious Diseases, Department of Medicine, Beth Israel Deaconess Medical Center, Department of Pediatrics, Boston Children's Hospital, Boston, Massachusetts

ALEXANDER J. McADAM, MD, PhD
Department of Laboratory Medicine, Medical Director, Infectious Diseases Diagnostic Laboratory, Boston Children's Hospital, Associate Professor of Pathology, Harvard Medical School, Boston, Massachusetts

ERIN McELVANIA, PhD, D(ABMM)
Department of Pathology and Laboratory Medicine, NorthShore University Health System, Evanston, Illinois

MARTHA H. McGEE, BS, MT(ASCP)
Director, McLendon Clinical Laboratories, UNC HealthCare, Chapel Hill, North Carolina

STEPHANIE L. MITCHELL, PhD, D(ABMM)
Assistant Professor, Department of Pathology, Director of Clinical Microbiology, UPMC Children's Hospital of Pittsburgh, University of Pittsburgh School of Medicine, Pittsburgh, Pennsylvania

DAVID R. PEAPER, MD, PhD
Department of Laboratory Medicine, VA Connecticut Health Care, Yale School of Medicine, New Haven, Connecticut

STEFAN RIEDEL, MD, PhD, D(ABMM), FCAP
Associate Professor, Department of Pathology, Harvard Medical School, Associate Medical Director, Clinical Microbiology Laboratories, Beth Israel Deaconess Medical Center, Boston, Massachusetts

PATRICIA J. SIMNER, PhD, D(ABMM)
Associate Professor of Pathology, Director of Bacteriology and Parasitology, Division of Medical Microbiology, Department of Pathology, Johns Hopkins School of Medicine, Baltimore, Maryland

KENNETH P. SMITH, PhD
Postdoctoral Fellow, Department of Pathology, Beth Israel Deaconess Medical Center, Harvard Medical School, Center for Life Science, Boston, Massachusetts

VINCENT H. TAM, PharmD
Departments of Pharmacy Practice and Translational Research, and Pharmacological and Pharmaceutical Sciences, University of Houston College of Pharmacy, Houston, Texas

RICHARD B. THOMSON Jr, PhD, D(ABMM), FAAM
Department of Pathology and Laboratory Medicine, NorthShore University Health System, Evanston, Illinois

AUDREY WANGER, PhD
Department of Pathology and Laboratory Medicine, University of Texas Health Science Center at Houston, Houston, Texas

Contents

> With emerging antimicrobial resistance, rapid antimicrobial susceptibility testing (AST) is needed to provide early definitive therapeutic guidance to optimize patient outcome. Genotypic methods are fast, but can identify only a subset of known resistance elements. Phenotypic methods determine clinically predictive minimal inhibitory concentrations and include very sensitive optical and biophysical methods to detect changes in replication or physiology of pathogens in response to antibiotics. For the potential of rapid AST to be fully realized, results must be linked with robust decision support solutions that will implement therapeutic changes in real time.

> Antibacterial combinations have long been used to accomplish a variety of therapeutic goals, including prevention of resistance and enhanced antimicrobial activity. In vitro synergy testing methods, including the checkerboard array, the time-kill study, diffusion assays, and pharmacokinetic/pharmacodynamic models, are used commonly in the research setting, but are not routinely performed in the clinical microbiology laboratory because of test complexity and uncertainty about their predictive value for patient outcomes. Optimized synergy testing techniques and better data on the relationship between in vitro results and clinical outcomes are needed to guide the rational use of antimicrobial combinations in the multidrug resistance era.

> The article discusses the environment of laboratory diagnostic bacteriology testing in several underresourced settings experienced by the author. The major global infectious diseases are usually managed with government or donor-supported systems, whereas basic laboratory testing for bacterial infections has no formal global programs. The causes of many of those diseases can be detected using simple manual bacteriologic methods available in most resource-limited environments; however, the challenges of building laboratory capacity in those settings are many. Positive and negative aspects of developing such capacities in selected locations are presented.

molecular methodology, emerging biomarkers, and informatics. We describe strengths, weaknesses, opportunities, and threats to the development of point-of-care diagnostics in the near (1–10 years) and more distant (10–20 years) future.

This article describes the current state of the art with regards to commercially available syndromic panels for blood stream infections, gastrointestinal pathogen detection, respiratory tract infections, and central nervous system infections, while providing a provocative and speculative look into the future of syndromic panel testing for infectious diseases.

Sepsis and pneumonia cause significant morbidity and mortality worldwide. Despite improvements in diagnostic methodologies for organism identification, the early recognition and further risk stratification of these infections can be challenging. Although traditional clinical scoring systems are beneficial for the management of sepsis and pneumonia, biomarkers supporting the diagnosis and management of these infectious diseases are needed. Many biomarkers have been identified and there is no lack of studies and meta-analyses assessing the utility of biomarkers. Focusing primarily on sepsis and pneumonia, this article discusses the most commonly used biomarkers for which clinical laboratory testing methods are available.

As a class, β-lactamase inhibitors have proved successful in extending the clinical utility of β-lactam antibiotics by circumventing β-lactamase–mediated resistance. However, the rapid evolution of these β-lactamases calls for a critical reevaluation of the relationships between susceptibility, drug exposures, and bacterial response. The existing paradigm for in vitro susceptibility testing and development of β-lactam/β-lactamase inhibitor combinations may not optimally facilitate clinical use. Thus, alternative approaches for pairing these combinations and evaluating in vitro susceptibility are needed to provide better guidance to clinicians.

Rapidly changing technology in the clinical microbiology laboratory requires a highly skilled workforce. The current clinical microbiology workforce is aging with a wave of retirements currently unfolding. Key competencies that will be needed for the next generation of microbiologists include strong analytical skills, adaptability, and the willingness to be life-long learners. Experiential learning is a key component of the initial learning environment for medical laboratory scientists and technicians. Continuing education in clinical microbiology must reflect the changes in technology whereby learners are more comfortable in an electronic learning environment, such as TED Talks and YouTube.

Infectious diseases by definition spread and therefore have impact beyond local hospitals and institutions where they occur. With increasingly complex and worrisome infectious disease evolution including emergence of multidrug resistance, regional, national, and international agencies and resources must work hand in hand with local clinical microbiology laboratories to address these global threats. Described are examples of such resources, both existing and aspirational, that will be needed to address the infectious disease challenges ahead. The authors comment on several instances of entrenched policy that are nonproductive and may be worthy of revision to address unmet needs in infectious disease diagnostics.

Pictorial Illustration

Clinical microbiology has advanced tremendously in the past 10 years. In this comic, the role of technology, the need for skilled microbiologists, and the meaning of progress in clinical microbiology are considered.

CLINICS IN LABORATORY MEDICINE

SERIES OF RELATED INTEREST

Surgical Pathology Clinics
Available at: https://www.surgpath.theclinics.com/

THE CLINICS ARE NOW AVAILABLE ONLINE!
Access your subscription at:
www.theclinics.com

Preface

Our Pathogens Are Not Standing Still and Neither Can We

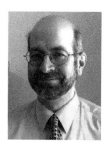

James E. Kirby, MD, D(ABMM)
Editor

In 1 or 2 generations, we have gone from a world in which there were no cures for most infections to a declaration that the war against infectious disease was won. That period of ephemeral confidence was followed by the inexorable march toward increasingly resistant pathogens that quickly learned to evade each new advance and our own race, sometimes successful, sometimes faltering, to produce new antimicrobials and vaccines.

As a society, in turn, we have disincentivized investment in new antimicrobials and have seen decades of relative stagnation in development. At the same time, advances in molecular, cellular, computational, and structural biology; medicinal chemistry, microbial epidemiology; and diagnostics have led to spectacular progress in prevention and treatment of viral, bacterial, and parasitic diseases. I consider clinical microbiology a lynchpin in these successes, and despite the challenges ahead, the current and future contributions of clinical microbiology as a discipline, highlighted in articles in this issue, leave me optimistic.

It is well to remember that advances in treating cancer and autoimmune disease are associated with prolonged, often profound periods of immunosuppression. Infections are almost inevitable. Therefore, at their foundation, modern medicine is predicated on being able to rapidly identify and successfully treat infectious diseases. These infections will occur in the context of a world where empiric treatment efficacy is far less predictable. Therefore, the clinical microbiology advances described in this issue will help sustain medical advances that depend on containing infectious diseases.

In the next 20 years, I see an increasingly more crowded, more mobile world where infectious diseases can spread quickly. Emergence and spread of multidrug-resistant, carbapenemase-producing Enterobacteriaceae and Ebola virus outbreaks are examples. I am also mindful of the unpredictability of pathogen evolution and their occasional lack of concern for the well-being of their hosts, for example, introduction of a

Clin Lab Med 39 (2019) xiii–xiv
https://doi.org/10.1016/j.cll.2019.06.001
0272-2712/19/© 2019 Published by Elsevier Inc.

myxovirus, which killed 99% of Australia's rabbit population.[1] Would there be a similar fate for humans without tools in hand to diagnose, treat, and preempt?

The articles in this issue describe a series of tools, applications, insights, and approaches to address the challenges ahead. I thank all the authors for their very insightful contributions, roughly divided into 3 categories. The first is technological: what new techniques are available to provide the fastest, most accurate, and impactful infectious disease diagnostics to our patients? From microfluids to next-generation sequencing to clever multiplex syndromic-based nucleic acid amplification panels. The second considers how we apply these advances (point of care, automation). The third considers larger issues of how to bring advances or even more basic clinical microbiology capabilities to all areas of the world, including the role of public health infrastructure to coordinate and leverage these efforts, and how to educate clinical microbiologists of the future. Regarding the last, I especially welcome the contributions from several authors who are clinical fellows, and who will soon assume leadership positions in clinical microbiology and related fields. I am also grateful for the pictorial representation of some of the dilemmas in clinical microbiology from the perspective of two of our major pathogens, who do not always see cocci to cocci with one another.

Reading the articles, I am struck by and thrilled with the level of innovation in our field. I look forward to the next 20 years of clinical microbiology.

James E. Kirby, MD, D(ABMM)
Department of Pathology
Beth Israel Deaconess Medical Center
330 Brookline Avenue–YA309
Boston MA 02215, USA

E-mail address:
jekirby@bidmc.harvard.edu

REFERENCE

1. Yong E. The next article in a viral arms race. The Atlantic. 2017. Available at: https://www.theatlantic.com/science/archive/2017/08/rabbit-virus-arms-race/536796/. Accessed April 6, 2019.

Rapid Susceptibility Testing Methods

Kenneth P. Smith, PhD[a], James E. Kirby, MD, D(ABMM)[b,c],*

KEYWORDS

- Rapid antimicrobial susceptibility testing • Antimicrobial resistance • Phenotypic
- Genotypic

KEY POINTS

- Emerging antimicrobial resistance makes empiric therapy unreliable. Therefore, rapid antimicrobial susceptibility testing (AST) will provide early, definitive therapeutic guidance to optimize patient outcome.
- Genotypic rapid AST methods are fast but can only identify what we know about. Phenotypic rapid AST methods provide a nuanced integrated assessment of resistance that can be used to pick the most active therapies.
- Early detection by phenotypic AST methods requires very sensitive technology, such as microscopic detection of replicating organisms, biophysical assessment, or signal amplification techniques.
- For the potential of rapid AST platforms to be fully realized, results must be linked with robust, autonomous decision support solutions that will implement therapeutic changes in real time.

INTRODUCTION

Antimicrobial susceptibility testing (AST) is a fundamental mission of the clinical microbiology laboratory. AST provides an in vitro measure of bacterial response to an antimicrobial agent that predicts therapeutic efficacy. Standard AST methods require isolated organisms and effectively take a day to perform. Thus, a minimum of 2 days is required to obtain susceptibility information from a clinical sample. With

Disclosure Statement: J.E. Kirby is a member of the Clinical Advisory Board of First Light Biosciences, Chelmsford, MA. TECAN (Morrisville, NC) provided an HP D300 digital dispenser and associated consumables used by JEK's research group during development of the MAST platform. Neither First Light nor TECAN had a role in article preparation or decision to publish.
[a] Department of Pathology, Beth Israel Deaconess Medical Center, Harvard Medical School, Center for Life Science, 3 Blackfan Circle-CLS624, Boston, MA 02115, USA; [b] Clinical Microbiology, Department of Pathology, Beth Israel Deaconess Medical Center, 330 Brookline Avenue-YA309, Boston, MA, USA; [c] Harvard Medical School, Boston, MA, USA
* Corresponding author. Department of Pathology, Beth Israel Deaconess Medical Center, 330 Brookline Avenue-YA309, Boston, MA.
E-mail address: jekirby@bidmc.harvard.edu

emerging resistance, this delay may lead to a prolonged AST gap during which patients are treated with suboptimal or ineffective therapy. Rapid AST methods are needed to close this gap. In this review, the authors summarize new and evolving approaches to rapid AST. Importantly, if a rapid AST method provides a timely result and no one is aware, the authors rhetorically query (akin to the proverbial fallen tree in the forest) whether it is truly rapid. Therefore, the authors suggest that rapid AST must go hand in hand with new decision support technology to enable an equally rapid therapeutic response.

FROM REFERENCE TO COMMERCIAL METHODS: CURRENT STATE

AST methods based on broth or agar dilution are used to determine the minimal inhibitory concentration (MIC), defined as the lowest concentration of antimicrobial inhibiting growth in vitro. Organizations such as the Clinical and Laboratory Standards Institute and the European Committee on Antimicrobial Susceptibility Testing, correlate MICs with pharmacokinetic/pharmacodynamics (PK/PD) studies and clinical outcome to derive categorical interpretive criteria (sensitive, resistant, and so forth) upon which antimicrobial therapeutic selections are made. The gold-standard dilution-based methods, broth macrodilution and microdilution and agar dilution, have remained relatively unchanged for greater than 40 years.[1]

These methods serve as reference comparators for clearance of all commercial AST testing systems. However, they are labor intensive and complex so they are rarely if ever performed outside a reference laboratory setting. Instead, most clinical laboratories use automated platforms for routine AST with generally comparable performance characteristics. AST may also be performed with commercially prepared broth dilution panels, or using antimicrobial disk or gradient strip diffusion methods. Practically, results from all of these methods are not available until the next day, and therapeutic corrections in response to results may be delayed even further. All of these methods require inoculation with isolated bacterial colonies, although direct testing of positive culture broth without colony isolation (decreasing turnaround by a day) has proven reasonably reliable using disk diffusion.[2]

WITH EMERGING ANTIMICROBIAL RESISTANCE, TIMELINESS BECOMES IMPORTANT

Until recently, predictable susceptibility profiles allowed for reliable selection of effective empiric antimicrobial therapy, making a 1- to 2-day AST gap clinically acceptable (**Fig. 1**). However, emerging antimicrobial resistance has led to a higher incidence of empiric therapy failure. In particular, for bloodstream infections, mortality correlates with the time needed to get patients on active therapy.[3] Delay may have less impact on localized infections such as uncomplicated cystitis and pyelonephritis.[4] Nevertheless, patients suffer in the short term from symptom prolongation and are at increased risk of complications while on suboptimal therapy.

Therefore, rapid AST will support several clinical goals. First, with emerging antimicrobial resistance, rapid AST will identify active therapy in time to optimize outcome.[5] Second, rapid AST will support antimicrobial stewardship goals by allowing timely transition from increasingly broad-spectrum regimens to pathogen-specific therapy. This narrowing of coverage reduces (1) exposure to potentially toxic broad-spectrum single and combination antimicrobial regimens[6,7]; (2) complications such as *Clostridiodes difficile* colitis; and (3) selection for antimicrobial-resistant pathogens in the patient's colonizing flora, a setup for future multidrug-resistant infection. Based on these considerations, rapid AST methods are not surprisingly an area of intense investigation.

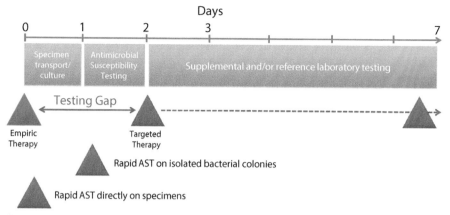

Fig. 1. Reducing the antimicrobial testing gap. Rapid AST will reduce the time between the start of empiric therapy and definitive therapy based on AST data by at least 1 day for methods that test isolated bacterial growth and by at least 2 days for methods that test primary specimens directly. Rapid AST data will allow life-saving therapeutic corrections and tailoring of therapy to foster stewardship goals and avoid complications from extended broad-spectrum empiric therapy.

RAPID SUSCEPTIBILITY LANDSCAPE OVERVIEW

There are 2 broad classes of AST technology: genotypic and phenotypic, each of which has advantages and disadvantages. The most impactful rapid susceptibility methods would yield results in a few hours. However, holistically, "rapid" must also take into account time required for all preanalytic and postanalytic components leading to therapeutic adjustments.

GENOTYPIC TESTING

Genotypic AST detects the presence of specific resistance genes, which may encode enzymes that degrade antibiotic (eg, β-lactamases), modify antibiotic target (eg, ribosomal methylases), or alter the target via mutation or substitution (eg, acquisition of penicillin-binding protein 2a by *Staphylococcus aureus*). Genotypic susceptibility testing can provide rapid results because neither growth nor metabolism is required for readout. Furthermore, genotypic testing, unlike traditional AST methods, can be performed directly on primary specimens and positive blood culture broth, greatly reducing time to diagnosis.

However, genotypic testing only detects what it is designed to detect, and conversely will not detect what is not yet known. In addition, it provides no information about penetrance, to what degree a resistance element is phenotypically expressed, and so may overcall resistance. For example, low levels of serine carbapenemase expression may result in carbapenem MICs (susceptible or intermediate) that should be treatable based on PK/PD considerations.[8,9] Of course, it may be argued whether phenotypic MICs are sufficiently reliable based on the steep inoculum effect observed at bacterial concentrations used for AST testing[10]; whether sufficient PK/PD exploration has been performed to justify use of carbapenems for carbapenem-producing strains, when other options are available; and thus, whether a more conservative approach based on gene detection is preferred.[10] However, it is certain that targeted genetic methods lack nuance.

THE GRAM-POSITIVE/NEGATIVE GENOTYPIC DIVIDE

The predictive value and utility of genotypic AST is strongest for gram-positive pathogens. Here, a relatively small number of resistance elements (mecA/C, vanA/B) contribute to the preponderance of phenotypically observed resistance to therapeutics of major interest.

However, the gram-positive, mecA target itself also illustrates the not necessarily apparent complexity of genotypic testing. The mecA gene exists within staphylococcal chromosomal cassette (SCCmec), a mobile genetic element that is heterogeneous.[11] Therefore, a large number of primer sets have been incorporated into nucleic acid amplification tests (NAATs) to ensure reliable detection. This is especially important because the clinical consequences of calling a methicillin-resistant blood isolate inappropriately susceptible to β-lactams can be devastating, that is, a switch to ineffective therapy for an aggressive infection. Furthermore, this genetic heterogeneity is not static. As an exemplar, emergence of mecC in S aureus led to missed detection of methicillin-resistant S aureus in mecA assays.[12] Therefore, microbial evolution necessitates vigilance and diagnostic product evolution with associated regulatory, technical, and economic hurdles, ultimately limiting NAAT assays to only the most common, relatively stable targets.

In contrast, gram-negative pathogens frequently exhibit resistance mechanisms that are polygenic and reflect combinatorial effects of permeability, efflux, target modification, enzymatic degradation, and potentially other mechanisms as well. For example, predicting how the hundreds of distinct β-lactamases, which may be expressed in different combinations and at different levels, would affect the MIC against a variety of β-lactam agents seems a daunting task. With this complexity, an inclusive, fully predictive assay may be an elusive goal.

Nevertheless, platforms that rapidly detect the presence or absence of high consequence resistance elements, such as KPC, VIM, IMP, OXA, and NDM carbapenemases, will allow therapeutic adjustment and/or potential reach for agents not typically used for empiric therapy. Genotypic resistance detection within syndromic panels is further discussed in Marc Roger Couturier and Jennifer Dien Bard's article, "Direct-from-Specimen Pathogen Identification: Evolution of Syndromic Panels," in this issue.

With total analytical times likely to trend under 10 minutes with advanced polymerase chain reaction techniques and related technologies, these types of panels will offer very rapid, targeted direction for a subset of pathogens and resistance types.[13] The potential application of whole genome sequencing for AST, the logical extreme of multiplexed genotypic testing, is reviewed in Stephanie L. Mitchell and Patricia J. Simner's article, "Next-Generation Sequencing from Strain Typing to Identification to Antimicrobial Susceptibility Prediction: Will It Supplant Traditional Methods in the Clinical Microbiology Laboratory, When and at What Cost?," in this issue.

CHALLENGES OF RAPID PHENOTYPIC ANTIMICROBIAL SUSCEPTIBILITY TESTING

A wide body of PK/PD data has been used to set categorical breakpoints based on phenotypic MICs determined by reference methods. Broadly, relation of pharmacokinetic profiles to phenotypic MIC predicts treatment efficacy based on well-established parameters that appear thus far agnostic to underlying resistance gene repertoire. For example, time over the MIC is predictive of a successful response to β-lactam therapy, reviewed in Henrietta Abodakpi and colleagues' article, "What the Clinical Microbiologist Should Know About PK/PD In The Era of Emerging Multidrug-Resistance: Beta-Lactam/Beta-Lactamase Inhibitor Combinations," in this issue. Therefore, rapid determination of the phenotypic MIC would provide significant value.

Currently, all reference AST methods are based on direct visual observation of an organism's response to antibiotics. The threshold for visual detection requires more than a 200-fold increase in bacterial numbers from the initial inoculum. Accordingly, such bulk growth AST assays require an extended incubation period (16–20 hours) to reach reliable detection thresholds.

Earlier assessment of growth is complicated by both biological and technical factors. A major biological factor is the "lag phase," during which organisms metabolically adapt to a new environment, but do not yet reproduce.[14] Measurements made before organisms exit this lag phase may result in erroneous categorization of organisms as antibiotic susceptible. Lag phase can last for 1 to 2 hours under optimal conditions and may be extended in the presence of stressors, including exposure to subinhibitory levels of antibiotics during MIC testing.[15]

Even during the active growth phase, genes required for antimicrobial resistance may take a finite time to be expressed. Furthermore, measurements may be confounded by altered morphology of organisms in the presence of antibiotics. For example, gram-negative cells exposed to inhibitory concentrations of β-lactams or fluoroquinolones form filaments,[16] potentially making it difficult to distinguish between increased volume and true replication.

Biological limitations notwithstanding, rapid phenotypic AST methods must detect organism growth and/or metabolism with very low organism burden. Therefore, the most significant requirement for rapid phenotypic AST is sufficiently sensitive measurement techniques. Several innovative technologies have emerged to address these challenges, broken down by general category in later discussion.

MICROSCOPY-BASED RAPID PHENOTYPIC ANTIMICROBIAL SUSCEPTIBILITY TESTING

The conceptually simplest way to determine whether an organism's replication is inhibited by an antibiotic is to count bacterial cell numbers by microscopy. However, such measurements are complicated by the need to confine bacteria to a focal plane within a sufficiently optically clear medium to allow microscopic image analysis. Several different strategies have been explored, including electrophoretic or centrifugal immobilization onto an adherent surface covered by liquid growth medium; inkjet printing of organisms onto a solid growth surface; or confinement to a microfluidic droplet or channel, several examples of which are discussed in turn. This list is not a comprehensive listing, but illustrates the diversity of approaches being pursued. The evolution and natural selection of the most propitious methods will play out over the next decades.

One commercialized system electrophoreses organisms from positive blood culture broth (presumably applicable to primary samples as well) onto a solid surface. An automated microscope records transition from individual organisms to microcolonies in the presence or absence of a panel of antibiotics. MICs are determined based on a machine-learning algorithm that evaluates growth effects of a single concentration of antibiotic during several hours of incubation. These extrapolated MICs have been reported to be accurate.[17]

Both the elegance and the complexity of this system are emblematic of the tradeoffs that must be reconciled as the field matures. For example, the existing one sample per shift per instrument throughput is a concern in high-volume laboratories. The underlying complexity also necessarily comes at a price that will not address the needs of resource limited (see Ellen Jo Baron's article, "Clinical Microbiology in Under-

Resourced Settings," in this issue for further discussion) and perhaps even not so resource limited settings as well.

The authors' own group is developing a technology that uses inkjet printing of pathogen and antibiotics onto a solidified Mueller-Hinton–based growth surface.[18] The system allows testing of any antimicrobial at any concentration at will using commercially available microplates, consumables, and reagents.[19] Automated microscopy is combined with a trained convolutional neural network–based algorithm to allow for highly automated MIC determination. Although still early in development, this system has shown greater than 95% agreement for testing standard quality-control strains with representative classes of antibiotics in a 2-hour time frame.[18] In its current form, it would need to be combined with a separate bacterial identification system, for example, matrix-assisted laser desorption time-of-flight mass spectrometry (MALDI-TOF), to allow appropriate interpretation. Another recently described microscopic technology follows growth of bacteria immobilized in agarose in a customized 96-well-plate format from positive blood culture broth with AST determinations in 4 hours.[20]

MICROSCOPY PLUS MICROFLUIDICS

A variety of microfluidic-based methods for AST have been described in which bacteria are confined within channels or nanodroplets and assayed by traditional or fluorescence microscopy.[21] Microfluidic devices are custom manufactured and may require pumping and sample loading methods that increase device complexity, cost, and scalability. However, implementation of microfluidics in infectious disease sample-to-answer NAATs suggests that these technologies can be successfully commercialized.

ALTERNATIVE OPTICAL DETECTION METHODS

A fundamental challenge for direct microscopy-based AST methods is the need for magnification (typically $\geq 400\times$), which demands relatively complex and potentially costly optics and automation (for example, an autofocus system coupled to a mechanized stage). In one alternative strategy, organisms from primary samples after exposure to antibiotic and an incubation phase are tethered to magnetic beads and labeled with fluorescence in situ hybridization probes unique for each species and then pulled by a magnet through a light blocking dye-cushion, thereby optically separating labeled bacteria from specimen matrix and unbound reporter.[22] Organisms are counted without magnification using a complementary metal-oxide semiconductor digital camera chip allowing species-specific quantitative analysis.

An alternative method uses forward laser light scatter, in a way similar to flow cytometry, but in bulk bacterial growth suspension. This biophysical bacterial enumeration method, already commercialized for quantifying bacteria in urine specimens, has been applied to direct AST on urine specimens and positive blood culture broth.[23,24]

SPECTROMETRY-BASED DETECTION

Raman spectroscopy–based methods rely on spectral scattering of an incident monochromatic laser beam to detect potentially very early physiologic changes in bacteria exposed to antibiotics and deposited on a solid surface for analysis.[25] To date, no Raman spectroscopy–based AST methods have been comprehensively evaluated, and the potential for cost-effective commercialization of these complex technologies remain unclear.

MALDI-TOF has become commonplace in the clinical microbiology laboratory as a qualitative technique for species identification. There has been some progress toward using peak intensity as a proxy for bacterial growth, which can in turn be applied to phenotypic AST.[26] However, to transition this technology into clinical practice, significant additional levels of automation will be required. Furthermore, applicability to direct specimen AST seems a steep hurdle, and the cost of underlying instrumentation will make deployment at point of care unfeasible. MALDI-TOF is discussed in more depth in Alexandra L. Bryson and colleagues' article, "MALDI-TOF: The Revolution in Progress," in this issue.

SIGNAL AMPLIFICATION

Detection of small numbers of bacteria can also be addressed through signal amplification techniques using either physical or molecular detection methods. For example, after standard incubation for several hours in a 384-well format, one platform uses robotics to introduce cationic, europium-cryptate-diamine chelate into microplates that nonspecifically coat and bind to natively anionic bacterial surfaces.[27] After a washing step to remove unbound chelate, time-resolved fluorescence signal from the chelate correlates with total bacterial surface area and accurately predicts MIC values.

Several strategies use nucleic acid amplification technology (NAAT) to quantify organism number or transcriptional activity and provide a much earlier readout of growth and viability than bulk growth assays.[28] A variation uses replication incompetent phage particles to introduce a reporter (eg, luciferase gene) into bacteria in a species-specific manner for both identification and AST. Luminescence, an ATP-dependent process, provides a proxy for bacterial viability. The technique is potentially applicable to direct testing of patient samples with low organism burden.[29] Notably, all of the signal amplification assays discussed are endpoint determinations with a fixed, single incubation time for analysis. These fixed determinations will need to confront lag time and resistance induction issues that can be more easily addressed by real-time phenotypic measures.

DECISION SUPPORT MUST GO HAND IN HAND WITH RAPID ANTIMICROBIAL SUSCEPTIBILITY TESTING IMPLEMENTATION

Faster AST results should lead to reduced morbidity and mortality, shorter hospital stays, and cost savings. However, in practice, several factors prevent full realization of these benefits. These factors include inadequate communication and therapeutic inertia, reluctance to switch from broad empiric broad-spectrum therapy, if active, to directed therapy.

These factors likely contribute to the less than impressive, but nevertheless instructive, findings in the rapid diagnostics literature. These studies primarily examined the impact of rapid diagnostic molecular testing performed on positive blood culture broth in comparison to traditional methods. They further focused almost exclusively on pathogen identification rather than rapid susceptibility testing, and therapeutic changes were primarily seen for gram-positive infections. However, two important lessons can still be distilled. First, even without AST guidance, there was significant improvement in time to effective therapy (5 hours) and reduced length of hospital stay (2.5 days).[30] Second, significant improvement in mortality was only demonstrated in the presence of an antimicrobial team on call to respond to "rapid data" and to assist in therapeutic adjustment. With some exceptions, it is doubtful that significant change in therapy would have been made in advance of classic AST for gram-negative pathogens. Therefore, the power of rapid AST is recognized but has not yet been fully demonstrated in the literature.[31]

Over the next 20 years, the number of therapeutic choices will certainly increase as will prevalence of antimicrobial resistance (**Fig. 2**). Therefore, the likely efficacy of empiric therapy will decrease. Furthermore, with increasing number of potential agents, new dosing strategies, and insights from personalized metabolomics, it will be more difficult for caregivers to master optimal use of these agents (optimal dosing, drug interactions, contraindications, and adjustments for disease conditions) and render timely, informed therapeutic decisions to take full advantage of rapid AST. However, such rapid therapeutic adjustments will become critical as empiric therapies become unreliable.

Ultimately, impact of rapid AST technologies will rely on care providers' willingness and ability to rapidly respond. It is clear that reliance on intervention from specially trained teams, although effective, is only a partial, resource-intensive, and not fully sustainable solution.

Therefore, the authors envision that rapid AST must be inextricably linked to a robust and ultimately autonomous decision support system. Such a system, which the authors call AST-ASSIST, will incorporate bundled orders, rapid identification, and susceptibility input; integration of the medical record; and automated flags and real-time therapeutic decisions or suggestions. Each component is discussed in turn, as outlined in **Fig. 3**. This system is designed to provide the most appropriate, timely antimicrobial therapy, while still enlisting direction from primary caregivers who are best aware of history, clinical considerations, and patient preferences not reflected in the medical record.

The authors envision leveraging clinicians' insights by allowing upfront decisions for multiple potential antimicrobial treatment options, or physician-ordered pathways (POPs). Specifically, when infection is suspected, a POP would consist of a single order, including both microbiological cultures and treatment. Constituted within this order would be broad-spectrum empiric antibiotics and a series of potential targeted antibiotic regimens that would be reflexed depending on definitive (rapid) AST results. Modifications to the POP would be suggested by AST-ASSIST through query of the

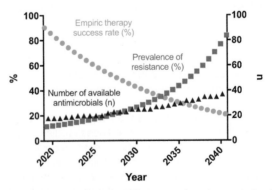

Fig. 2. Loss of reliable empiric therapy. Over the next 2 decades, antimicrobial resistance will increase significantly. The number of available antimicrobials will also increase, but not at the same pace. As a result, the likelihood that any given empiric therapy will be effective will decrease. Therefore, rapid AST will become increasingly necessary to ensure patients are on active therapy in time to make a difference.

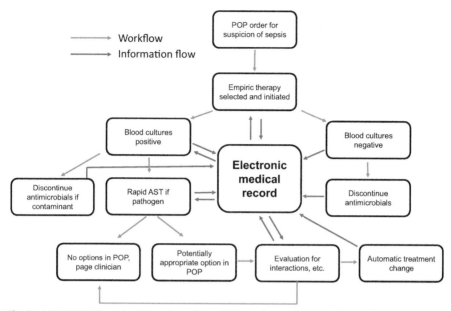

Fig. 3. AST-ASSIST. Rapid AST is only truly rapid if results can be acted on quickly. To this end, the authors envision a decision support system, AST-ASSIST, that will leverage use of POPs, which contains instructions for initial empiric antibiotics and options for reflexed directed antimicrobial therapy populated based on patient medical and microbiological history and local antibiogram. AST-ASSIST will implement therapeutic changes included within the POP based on organism identity and rapid AST results through interface with pharmacy and nursing systems and/or notify clinicians through pager or text message for additional timely input as needed.

electronic medical record (EMR) to consider patient allergies, interacting medications, underlying medical conditions, laboratory values (creatinine, liver function tests, cytopenias), and potential for resistance based on a current antibiogram, prior cultures, clinical service, and length and history of hospitalizations.

If organisms were detected, they would be subject to rapid antimicrobial identification and susceptibility testing using fully interfaced instrumentation. Therefore, data would be available in real time in the EMR. The authors envision that AST-ASSIST middleware would evaluate updated microbiological, laboratory, and clinical data from the medical record in real time to detect relevant changes since the original POP. For example, it would identify contraindications not detected in the initial POP evaluation, such as interactions with recently instituted therapies. If an appropriate targeted antimicrobial were initially included in the POP, an automatic update to pharmacy and nursing records would result in immediate change in therapy. If appropriate therapy were not included in the POP, clinicians would be alerted by pager/text message with a recommendation for an appropriate antimicrobial.

As an example of this process, if a patient were suspected to have sepsis, a POP would include blood cultures and specify empiric vancomycin/piperacillin-tazobactam as a broad-spectrum antimicrobial regimen based on the local antibiogram and patient history. If methicillin-susceptible *S aureus* were isolated, the AST-ASSIST system would evaluate the POP for optimal targeted therapy. If no contraindications were found, coverage would automatically be narrowed to a β-lactam, such as cefazolin, at the next dose, thereby minimizing all possible delay. However, if coagulase-negative staphylococci were isolated, the EMR would be automatically queried for previous positive cultures, elevated white cell count, fever, and biomarkers, such as procalcitonin (see Stefan Riedel's article, "Predicting Bacterial versus Viral Infection, or None of the Above: Current and Future Prospects of Biomarkers," in this issue), and lactate levels to predict the probability of a true infection versus contamination. Depending on the results and what was defined in the POP order, therapy may be stopped or the clinician paged to intervene.

Alternatively, if a carbapenem-resistant Enterobacteriaceae expressing a serine carbapenemase (with an MIC = 16 μg/mL by a phenotypic method) were isolated, an alert would be sent to nursing staff and pharmacy for immediate dosing of an appropriate active agent, for example, plazomicin, ceftazidime-avibactam, or meropenem-vaborbactam. Here, dose optimization of active agents may be particularly important owing to inherent toxicity or desire to optimize drug exposure based on PK/PD principles. Therefore, AST-ASSIST dosing algorithms would take into account body mass index, liver and kidney function, genetic metabolic knowledge, drug interactions with other onboard therapies, specific MIC of organism, and known PK/PD relationships to optimize dose and dosing frequency for particular agents, as applicable.

SUMMARY

Rapid AST represents a critical component in addressing the challenges posed by emerging antimicrobial resistance. A variety of phenotypic and genotypic methods are already Food and Drug Administration cleared or in development that promise to reduce the time to definitive AST results from days to hours. However, to optimize impact, those results must be shared with and acted on by health care providers *just as rapidly*. Therefore, rapid AST must be supported by a robust laboratory information system, EMR, and decision support infrastructure (POPs and AST-ASSIST). The authors look forward to fully integrated rapid AST systems and the advantages they will provide at all levels our health care system.

ACKNOWLEDGMENTS

Based on space limitations, it was not possible for the authors to reference and cite all of the relevant literature in the rapidly growing rapid AST field. They apologize to authors, scientists, and companies, large and small, whose innovative and important work could not specifically be identified in this review. The authors have purposely not mentioned the name of commercialized products to keep the focus on underlying principles. K.P.S. and J.E.K. were supported by the National Institute of Allergy and Infectious Diseases of the National Institutes of Health under award numbers F32AI124590, and R21AI130434, respectively. The content is solely the responsibility of the authors and does not necessarily represent the official views of the National Institutes of Health.

REFERENCES

1. Brennan-Krohn T, Smith KP, Kirby JE. The poisoned well: enhancing the predictive value of antimicrobial susceptibility testing in the era of multidrug resistance. J Clin Microbiol 2017;55(8):2304–8.
2. Chandrasekaran S, Abbott A, Campeau S, et al. Direct-from-blood-culture disk diffusion to determine antimicrobial susceptibility of gram-negative bacteria: preliminary report from the Clinical and Laboratory Standards Institute methods development and standardization working group. J Clin Microbiol 2018;56(3).

3. Rhodes A, Evans LE, Alhazzani W, et al. Surviving sepsis campaign: international guidelines for management of sepsis and septic shock: 2016. Intensive Care Med 2017;43(3):304–77.
4. Eliakim-Raz N, Babitch T, Shaw E, et al. Risk factors for treatment failure and mortality among hospitalized patients with complicated urinary tract infection: a multi-center retrospective cohort study (RESCUING Study Group). Clin Infect Dis 2019; 68(1):29–36.
5. Liu VX, Fielding-Singh V, Greene JD, et al. The timing of early antibiotics and hospital mortality in sepsis. Am J Respir Crit Care Med 2017;196(7):856–63.
6. Mullins BP, Kramer CJ, Bartel BJ, et al. Comparison of the nephrotoxicity of vancomycin in combination with cefepime, meropenem, or piperacillin/tazobactam: a prospective, multicenter study. Ann Pharmacother 2018;52(7):639–44.
7. Rutter WC, Cox JN, Martin CA, et al. Nephrotoxicity during vancomycin therapy in combination with piperacillin-tazobactam or cefepime. Antimicrob Agents Chemother 2017;61(2).
8. Tamma PD, Huang Y, Opene BN, et al. Determining the optimal carbapenem MIC that distinguishes carbapenemase-producing and non-carbapenemase-producing carbapenem-resistant enterobacteriaceae. Antimicrob Agents Chemother 2016;60(10):6425–9.
9. Neuner EA, Gallagher JC. Pharmacodynamic and pharmacokinetic considerations in the treatment of critically ill patients infected with carbapenem-resistant Enterobacteriaceae. Virulence 2017;8(4):440–52.
10. Smith KP, Kirby JE. The inoculum effect in the era of multidrug resistance: minor differences in inoculum have dramatic effect on MIC determination. Antimicrob Agents Chemother 2018;62(8).
11. Becker K, Ballhausen B, Kock R, et al. Methicillin resistance in Staphylococcus isolates: the "mec alphabet" with specific consideration of mecC, a mec homolog associated with zoonotic S. aureus lineages. Int J Med Microbiol 2014;304(7): 794–804.
12. Lee GH, Pang S, Coombs GW. Misidentification of Staphylococcus aureus by the Cepheid Xpert MRSA/SA BC assay due to deletions in the spa gene. J Clin Microbiol 2018;56(7).
13. Farrar JS, Wittwer CT. Extreme PCR: efficient and specific DNA amplification in 15-60 seconds. Clin Chem 2015;61(1):145–53.
14. Rolfe MD, Rice CJ, Lucchini S, et al. Lag phase is a distinct growth phase that prepares bacteria for exponential growth and involves transient metal accumulation. J Bacteriol 2012;194(3):686–701.
15. van Belkum A, Dunne WM Jr. Next-generation antimicrobial susceptibility testing. J Clin Microbiol 2013;51(7):2018–24.
16. Lorian V, Ernst J, Amaral L. The post-antibiotic effect defined by bacterial morphology. J Antimicrob Chemother 1989;23(4):485–91.
17. Pancholi P, Carroll KC, Buchan BW, et al. Multicenter evaluation of the accelerate PhenoTest BC kit for rapid identification and phenotypic antimicrobial susceptibility testing using morphokinetic cellular analysis. J Clin Microbiol 2018;56(4).
18. Smith KP, Richmond DL, Brennan-Krohn T, et al. Development of MAST: a microscopy-based antimicrobial susceptibility testing platform. SLAS Technol 2017;22(6):662–74.
19. Smith KP, Kirby JE. Verification of an automated, digital dispensing platform for at-will broth microdilution-based antimicrobial susceptibility testing. J Clin Microbiol 2016;54(9):2288–93.

20. Choi J, Jeong HY, Lee GY, et al. Direct, rapid antimicrobial susceptibility test from positive blood cultures based on microscopic imaging analysis. Sci Rep 2017; 7(1):1148.
21. Campbell J, McBeth C, Kalashnikov M, et al. Microfluidic advances in phenotypic antibiotic susceptibility testing. Biomed Microdevices 2016;18(6):103.
22. Gite S, Archambault D, Cappillino MP, et al. A rapid, accurate, single molecule counting method detects clostridium difficile toxin B in stool samples. Sci Rep 2018;8(1):8364.
23. Idelevich EA, Hoy M, Knaack D, et al. Direct determination of carbapenem-resistant Enterobacteriaceae and Pseudomonas aeruginosa from positive blood cultures using laser scattering technology. Int J Antimicrob Agents 2018;51(2): 221–6.
24. Montgomery S, Roman K, Ngyuen L, et al. Prospective evaluation of light scatter technology paired with matrix-assisted laser desorption ionization-time of flight mass spectrometry for rapid diagnosis of urinary tract infections. J Clin Microbiol 2017;55(6):1802–11.
25. Novelli-Rousseau A, Espagnon I, Filiputti D, et al. Culture-free antibiotic-susceptibility determination from single-bacterium Raman spectra. Sci Rep 2018;8(1):3957.
26. Jung JS, Hamacher C, Gross B, et al. Evaluation of a semiquantitative matrix-assisted laser desorption ionization-time of flight mass spectrometry method for rapid antimicrobial susceptibility testing of positive blood cultures. J Clin Microbiol 2016;54(11):2820–4.
27. Flentie K, Spears BR, Chen F, et al. Microplate-based surface area assay for rapid phenotypic antibiotic susceptibility testing. Sci Rep 2019;9(1):237.
28. Andini N, Hu A, Zhou L, et al. A "culture" shift: broad bacterial detection, identification, and antimicrobial susceptibility testing directly from whole blood. Clin Chem 2018;64(10):1453–62.
29. Roche gobbles Smarticles. Nat Biotechnol 2015;33(10):1012.
30. Timbrook TT, Morton JB, McConeghy KW, et al. The effect of molecular rapid diagnostic testing on clinical outcomes in bloodstream infections: a systematic review and meta-analysis. Clin Infect Dis 2017;64(1):15–23.
31. Henig O, Kaye KS, Chandramohan S, et al. The hypothetical impact of accelerate pheno on time to effective therapy and time to definitive therapy for bloodstream infections due to drug-resistant gram-negative bacilli. Antimicrob Agents Chemother 2019;63(3) [pii:e01477-18].

When One Drug Is Not Enough

Context, Methodology, and Future Prospects in Antibacterial Synergy Testing

Thea Brennan-Krohn, MD, D(ABMM)[a,b],
James E. Kirby, MD, D(ABMM)[c,*]

KEYWORDS

- Antimicrobial synergy • Synergy testing • Antimicrobial susceptibility testing
- Antimicrobial resistance • Checkerboard array • Time-kill assay
- Hollow fiber infection model

KEY POINTS

- Antibacterial combinations are used in clinical practice to accomplish a variety of therapeutic goals, including prevention of resistance and enhanced antimicrobial activity.
- The most common types of synergy testing are the checkerboard array assay, the time-kill study, diffusion assays, and pharmacokinetic/pharmacodynamic models (eg, hollow fiber infection model).
- Antibacterial synergy testing is not routinely performed in the clinical microbiology laboratory because of test complexity and uncertainty about the predictive value of synergy testing results for patient outcomes.
- Optimized synergy testing techniques and better data on the relationship between in vitro synergy results and clinical outcomes are needed to guide rational use of antimicrobial combinations in the multidrug resistance era.

Disclosure Statement: TECAN (Morrisville, NC) provided an HP D300 digital dispenser and associated consumables for use by JEK's research group. Tecan had no role in article preparation or decision to publish.
Funding: Dr. T. Brennan-Krohn's synergy research is supported by a National Institute of Allergy and Infectious Diseases career development award (1K08AI132716).

[a] Department of Pathology, Beth Israel Deaconess Medical Center, Harvard Medical School, 3 Blackfan Circle - CLS0624, Boston, MA 02115, USA; [b] Division of Infectious Diseases, Boston Children's Hospital, Harvard Medical School, 300 Longwood Avenue, Boston, MA 02115, USA; [c] Department of Pathology, Beth Israel Deaconess Medical Center, Harvard Medical School, 330 Brookline Avenue - YA309, Boston, MA 02215, USA
* Corresponding author.
E-mail address: jekirby@bidmc.harvard.edu

Clin Lab Med 39 (2019) 345–358
https://doi.org/10.1016/j.cll.2019.04.002
0272-2712/19/© 2019 Elsevier Inc. All rights reserved.

INTRODUCTION

Combination antibacterial therapy dates back to the early antibiotic era[1] and remains a common practice today. Some combinations have been widely used for decades, their clinical usefulness is well-supported by clinical outcomes data, whereas others have only recently been described in in vitro studies. A number of different techniques are used in the laboratory to test for synergistic activity in drug combinations. To understand the usefulness and limitations of these testing methods, we evaluate them in the context of the mechanisms they are designed to test and the various clinical rationales for antibacterial combination therapy.

MECHANISMS OF COMBINATION ANTIBIOTIC ACTIVITY

To make sense of synergy testing methods, it is essential to understand the mechanisms by which antibiotics can work when used in combination. There are 2 main conceptual reasons for using drugs in combination. The first is to prevent the emergence of resistance to any individual drug during treatment. Regimens used to prevent resistance are discussed briefly in Prevention of Resistance, in the context of *Mycobacterium tuberculosis*, but are not otherwise a primary focus in this review, because they do not rely on synergy in the sense of enhanced combinatorial activity, and their efficacy is not evaluated using synergy testing. The other reason to use 2 or more antibiotics together is that some drugs, in combination, exhibit activity that is greater than would be expected through simple additive activity; in other words, they are synergistic.

Prevention of Resistance

Discovered in 1943, streptomycin was the first drug in history with activity against *M tuberculosis*,[1,2] an ancient and deadly disease that has plagued humankind for thousands of years.[3] But it soon became apparent that *M tuberculosis* isolates from patients treated with streptomycin alone developed resistance to the drug during therapy[4]; only when multiple antituberculosis drugs were used in combination could resistance to any one of the agents reliably be prevented during the prolonged treatment courses required to cure tuberculosis.[1] Today, the standard initial regimen for drug-susceptible *M tuberculosis* isolates is a combination of 4 drugs: isoniazid, rifampin, ethambutol, and pyrazinamide.[5] Such multidrug regimens are essential for effective treatment because *M tuberculosis* develops resistance to each of these drugs relatively simply, through spontaneous chromosomal mutations.[6] As a result, during a standard course of tuberculosis therapy, which lasts at least 6 months,[5] the chance of an organism developing resistance to a drug used as monotherapy may be as high as 100%,[7] whereas the likelihood of an organism simultaneously developing resistance to 4 drugs is vanishingly small.

Enhanced Activity

Most bacterial pathogens do not develop resistance to antibiotics in as simple a manner as *M tuberculosis*,[8] and the use of combination regimens has not been shown to be an effective method for the prevention of resistance in organisms such as *Enterobacteriaceae*.[9] Instead, the primary rationale for the use of combination regimens in most bacterial pathogens is to overcome an existing resistance mechanism or to improve the activity of one or both agents[10] (**Table 1**).

SYNERGY TESTING METHODS

Several different methods are commonly used to test for synergy. These methods do not always yield identical results,[31–33] but determining which is most reliable is challenging,

Table 1
Mechanisms of synergistic antibacterial activity

Mechanism	Example(s)	Explanation	Clinical Testing Method
Inhibition of sequential steps in a biosynthetic pathway	Sulfamethoxazole + trimethoprim	Sulfamethoxazole and trimethoprim act synergistically[11] by inhibiting different steps in the production by bacteria of tetrahydrofolic acid, a key component in numerous bacterial biosynthetic processes.[12]	Drugs tested as a combination using standard AST
Inhibition of resistance mechanisms	Ampicillin-sulbactam, ceftazidime-avibactam	A β-lactam antibiotic combined with a β-lactamase inhibitor that protects the antibiotic from destruction by bacterial β-lactamase enzymes.[13]	Drugs tested as a combination using standard AST
Increased entry into the bacterial cell	Ampicillin or vancomycin + gentamicin for Enterococcus	Aminoglycosides (eg, gentamicin) are clinically ineffective against Enterococcus species owing to limited ability to enter the bacterial cell at in vivo concentrations. When given with an enterococcal cell wall-active drug (eg, ampicillin, vancomycin), gentamicin uptake is increased and its concentration at the ribosomal target reaches levels necessary for activity.[15]	High-level aminoglycoside resistance testing
	Colistin + drugs with limited ability to cross the outer membrane (eg, linezolid)[14]	Colistin and related compounds permeabilize the outer membrane of gram-negative bacteria. In vitro synergy between these agents and antibiotics that are not normally active against gram-negative bacteria[14,16,17] is believed to result from increased entry into the cell.[16]	Not performed

(continued on next page)

Table 1
(continued)

Mechanism	Example(s)	Explanation	Clinical Testing Method
Double β-lactam therapy for *Enterococcus*	Ampicillin + ceftriaxone for enterococcal endocarditis[18]	Complete saturation of nonessential penicillin-binding proteins by cephalosporins, which are ineffective against enterococci as monotherapy, in combination with partial saturation of essential penicillin-binding proteins by ampicillin, is believed to be mechanism of synergy.[19]	Not performed
Enhancement of biofilm activity	Addition of rifampin to regimens for staphylococcal prosthetic material infections (including prosthetic valve endocarditis)[20,21]	Rifampin, an inhibitor of bacterial DNA-dependent RNA polymerase, is almost never used as monotherapy because most bacteria rapidly develop resistance during therapy.[22] However, it is particularly active against biofilms and is often used for this purpose in combination with other drugs.	Not performed (*Staphylococcus* species tested for rifampin susceptibility by standard AST)
Unknown mechanisms	Amikacin + doripenem for carbapenemase-producing *Klebsiella pneumoniae*[23] Meropenem + levofloxacin for *Pseudomonas aeruginosa*[24] Fosfomycin + daptomycin for vancomycin-resistant *Enterococcus faecium*[25]	Using in vitro synergy methods and animal models, numerous antibiotic combinations have been tested against multidrug-resistant pathogens for which few standard treatment options exist, such as carbapenem-resistant Enterobacteriaceae,[23,26,27] *Pseudomonas aeruginosa*,[24,28] *Acinetobacter baumannii*,[29] and vancomycin-resistant enterococci.[25,30] Few studies have evaluated synergy mechanisms for these combinations.	Not performed

because there is no established gold-standard synergy reference method. An ideal technique would consistently predict treatment outcomes, but to date there have been few comparisons of in vitro synergy testing data with clinical outcomes; furthermore, different methods may work best for different organisms or drugs.[34]

Checkerboard Array

The checkerboard array method is an adaptation of standard broth-based minimal inhibitory concentration (MIC) testing. As such, it can assess the inhibition of bacterial growth, but does not provide information on bacterial killing.[35] The array is typically created in a 96-well microtiter plate, with each well containing a standardized bacterial inoculum and appropriate concentrations of antibiotics,[35] although adaptations using automated dispensing and smaller volumes have been described.[27] A typical checkerboard array layout is shown in **Fig. 1**. Microplates are examined for evidence of growth after incubation under standard antimicrobial susceptibility testing (AST) conditions.[36]

The results of a checkerboard array synergy assay are evaluated by calculating the fractional inhibitory concentration (FIC) index. In a well in which growth is inhibited, the FIC of each drug is determined by dividing the concentration of the drug in that well by the MIC of that drug alone.[35] The FIC index is the sum of the FIC values of 2 drugs in a

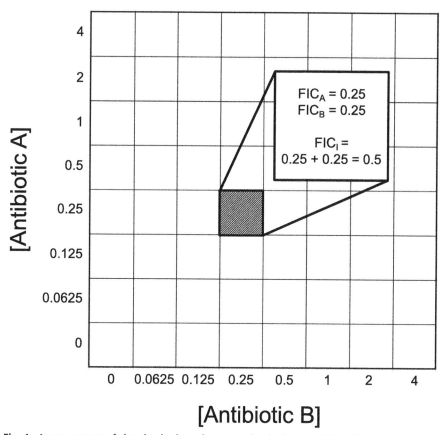

Fig. 1. Arrangement of the checkerboard array and calculation of the FIC_I. Antibiotic concentrations are expressed as multiples of the MIC. FIC, fractional inhibitory concentration; FIC_I, FIC index; FIC_A, FIC of antibiotic A; FIC_B, FIC of antibiotic B.

well. An FIC index of 0.5 or less is considered synergistic, whereas an FIC index of greater than 4.0 is antagonistic and intermediate values are considered to show no interaction.[37] It should be noted that to meet the definition of synergy, each drug must be present at less than one-half of its MIC. This definition reflects the expected variability of ± 1 two-fold dilution in single-agent MIC testing[38]: an FIC index of 1 could simply result from both drugs demonstrating inhibition at one-half their respective MICs by chance. Although the FIC index is the most common measure of synergy in the checkerboard array, other models have been developed.[39] In addition, the checkerboard array can be used to test more than 2 drugs at once,[40,41] although this method quickly becomes impractical unless limited concentration ranges are used for 1 or more of the drugs being tested.

Diffusion-Based Methods

Like the checkerboard array, diffusion-based synergy methods provide information about bacterial inhibition, but not about killing. Disk diffusion synergy testing is based on the principle of disk diffusion AST, in which a paper disk impregnated with the antibiotic of interest is placed on a lawn of bacteria on an agar plate. The drug diffuses through the agar and the diameter of the zone of bacterial clearance around the disk is measured after incubation and compared with established breakpoint tables to determine whether the organism is susceptible to the drug.[36,42] When this method is adapted for synergy testing, disks containing 2 different drugs are placed on a plate; if there is enhanced clearance or bridging between the 2 zones, the combination is considered synergistic, whereas if there is decreased clearance between the 2 zones, it is considered antagonistic.[43,44] Although this method is relatively simple to perform, it is not described often in the literature, perhaps because of concerns about subjectivity and a lack of established data.[10,43,45]

Antibiotic gradient diffusion strips work by a similar principle, except that the gradient of drug in the strip allows for the determination of an MIC value based on the point at which the ellipse of growth inhibition intersects with the strip.[46] Several methods for gradient strip synergy testing have been described, including the placement of strips at a right angle intersecting at the point of their relative MICs[33] and placing a strip containing 1 drug onto the agar in a location on which a strip containing the other drug had diffused before being removed.[47] The concentration at which each drug inhibits growth in the combination configuration is assessed after incubation, and these values are used to calculate an FIC index.[33,47]

Time-Kill Assay

The time-kill synergy assay is more labor intensive than the checkerboard array, and final results, which depend on the growth of bacterial samples for quantification, are delayed by a day compared with the checkerboard array. However, time-kill assays provide information not only on synergy, but also on the time course of bacterial growth and on bactericidal activity. In a time-kill synergy study, bacteria are incubated in liquid culture tubes under the following conditions: each antibiotic alone at a given concentration, the 2 antibiotics in combination at the same concentrations, and an antibiotic-free growth control.[48] Aliquots are removed from each tube for colony enumeration at the beginning of the experiment, at interval time points, and at 24 hours. If the colony count at 24 hours from the combination tube is 2 $\log_{10}$ or more less than the count from the tube containing the most active drug alone, the combination is synergistic.[49] If the colony count at 24 hours from the combination tube is 3 $\log_{10}$ or more less than the starting inoculum, then the combination is also bactericidal.[49]

It should be noted that the nature of the assessment of synergy is different in time-kill and checkerboard array studies. The time-kill study compares the same concentrations of antibiotic together and separately and evaluates whether the combination is more effective at 24 hours than either individual drug. By contrast, because the checkerboard array has a binary outcome measure (inhibition of bacterial growth as detected by the absence of visually apparent turbidity), it can only assess whether a given concentration combination is effective or not. A checkerboard array study answers the question, "By how much can drug concentrations can be reduced while still inhibiting growth?", whereas a time-kill study answers the question, "How much more effective is the combination than its constituent drugs?"

In Vitro Pharmacokinetic/Pharmacodynamic Models

In vitro pharmacokinetic/pharmacodynamic (PK/PD) models differ from other synergy assays in that antibiotic concentrations can be varied over time, mimicking tissue drug concentrations during antibiotic therapy and allowing for the simulation and comparison of different dosing regimens.[50] One of the most widely adopted PK/PD systems is the hollow-fiber infection model.[51–53] The hollow-fiber infection model includes a central compartment, representing the circulatory system, from which media containing varying concentrations of antibiotics is pumped continuously through semipermeable fibers in a capillary unit similar to a dialysis cartridge. The antibiotic diffuses through pores in the fibers into the peripheral compartment, which is inoculated with bacteria to represent a site of infection. Because bacteria are too small to pass through the pores, antibiotic concentrations can be changed without artificially changing the bacterial concentration. In addition, bacterial waste products can diffuse out through the pores, allowing for experimental durations of 2 weeks or more.[54] Such durations facilitate evaluation of the emergence of resistance during treatment.[55]

Animal Models

Although in vitro PK/PD models can mimic in vivo drug concentrations, there are features of in vivo infection, such as immune response and tissue environment, that cannot be fully replicated in artificial systems. Animal infection models, usually in mice, allow for synergy testing in a living organism of different types of infection, including thigh infection,[56] sepsis,[57] and pneumonia.[23] The significant physiologic differences that exist between model organisms and humans must be accounted for to the extent possible in these models, for example, by inhibiting murine renal function to mimic human drug metabolism[58] or inducing neutropenia to increase susceptibility to infection.[59]

SYNERGY TESTING IN THE CLINICAL MICROBIOLOGY LABORATORY

It is notable, given this variety of well-established methods, that synergy testing is not routinely performed on organisms from patient samples in the clinical microbiology laboratory. There are 2 reasons for this. First, most synergy methods are too labor intensive to be incorporated into the clinical laboratory workflow. Second, as is discussed in more in the section Clinical relevance of in vitro synergy testing results, there is considerable debate about the direct clinical applicability of synergy testing results, and interpretive criteria for synergy testing have not been adopted by the Clinical and Laboratory Standards Institute.

For a few well-established combinations with known mechanisms of synergy, however, standardized susceptibility testing methods with published interpretive criteria allow the clinical laboratory to assess the activity of the combination without performing a full synergy assay.[36] To test for acquired high-level aminoglycoside resistance, which is the primary mechanism of resistance to synergy between an aminoglycoside and a cell wall-active agent in *Enterococcus* species,[60] enterococci are exposed to very high levels of gentamicin (500 μg/mL) or streptomycin (1000 μg/mL).[36] Isolates with high-level aminoglycoside resistance are not inhibited by these concentrations, and such resistance predicts a lack of synergistic aminoglycoside activity against the isolate.[61] Most drugs that are used together for synergy, including β-lactam–β-lactamase inhibitor combinations and trimethoprim–sulfamethoxazole, are manufactured and administered to patients as combination products at fixed ratios,[11,13] and the laboratory simply tests these combinations using standard AST methods.

CLINICAL RELEVANCE OF IN VITRO SYNERGY TESTING RESULTS

A few commonly used drug combinations, including β-lactam–β-lactamase inhibitor combinations and trimethoprim–sulfamethoxazole, have been investigated in clinical studies, and their efficacy and advantages over single-agent therapy for appropriate infections have been well-established.[62,63] However, although dozens of different drug combinations have been tested in vitro against various different species of bacteria,[64,65] there remains uncertainty about the clinical relevance of these results. Combinations often seem to be synergistic against some isolates and not others,[66,67] but it is unclear whether this is due to variable efficacy of the combination from one strain to another, in which case testing of individual patient isolates might be indicated, or to variability in methods or techniques, in which case method standardization and development of more robust synergy testing techniques may be required. At the heart of the uncertainty about clinical applicability of synergy testing lies the paucity of data incorporating both in vitro and clinical data from the same isolates. With a few exceptions in the form of case reports and small series,[52,68–70] most clinical studies are retrospective investigations that do not include in vitro synergy data[71,72]; as a result, it is impossible to know whether such results could have predicted either the overall efficacy of the combination or its usefulness for specific patients.

One randomized, double-blind, controlled trial has been performed to evaluate the effect on patient outcomes of combination antibiotic testing to guide drug selection.[73] This study compared outcomes in patients with cystic fibrosis treated with antibiotic regimens selected based on in vitro multiple combination bactericidal antibiotic testing with those treated with regimens selected based on standard AST. The authors found no difference in time to next pulmonary exacerbation between the 2 treatment groups. Possible explanations for the lack of benefit from combination testing in this study include limitations in the applicability of in vitro AST results for isolates from patients with cystic fibrosis and the fact that the susceptibility of many of the isolates to different combination regimens had changed from the time of combination testing to the time of treatment.[74,75] It is important to note that multiple combination bactericidal antibiotic testing lacks one of the key characteristics of the synergy testing methods described earlier: it does not compare the activity of a combination to the activity of its constituent components.[73] In multiple combination bactericidal antibiotic testing, clinically relevant concentrations of antibiotics are combined and incubated with the bacterial isolate, and if no visible turbidity is detected after a fixed period of incubation, a colony count is performed to assess for bactericidal activity. However, if one of the drugs in a combination is bactericidal on its own, then it is not clear that improved activity would be expected from the use of a bactericidal combination that includes it.

Furthermore, even patients in this trial who were randomized to treatment based on standard AST still received drugs that had showed inhibitory activity in vitro. It seems likely that synergy testing may turn out to be most useful not in incrementally improving outcomes of patients for whom standard therapeutic options exist, but in identifying effective salvage therapy regimens for patients infected with panresistant isolates[52,55] for which treatments do not otherwise exist.

THE FUTURE OF SYNERGY TESTING

As options for the treatment of increasingly resistant bacteria dwindle, synergistic anti-microbial regimens that rescue the activity of existing drugs offer the prospect of significantly expanded treatment options. However, more high-quality data are needed to determine which combinations are clinically effective for which organisms and to establish evidence-based standards for performing and interpreting synergy testing in the clinical laboratory. Progress along several axes will be essential to this process.

Clinical Trials Incorporating In Vitro Synergy Data

As discussed elsewhere in this article, very few clinical trials that compare combination therapy to monotherapy (or different combination regimens to each other) have included in vitro synergy testing. Most such clinical studies show mixed outcomes or demonstrate no overall benefit from combination therapy.[9,72] However, if only a subset of bacterial isolates are susceptible to a combination (just as only some isolates are susceptible to any given antibiotic), then these trials, which presumably include patients infected with both synergy-susceptible and synergy-nonsusceptible strains with no information about which is which, may show no overall effect, even if the combination would have been beneficial for some patients. Only if future clinical trials test patient isolates for in vitro synergy will it be possible to establish a relationship between in vitro synergy results and clinical outcomes.

Simpler Synergy Testing Methods

The technical complexity of synergy testing currently limits its inclusion in clinical trials, particularly in retrospective studies that rely on data collected during routine clinical care. Furthermore, because on-demand synergy testing is not available clinically for standard bacterial pathogens, the usefulness of synergy testing-based combination therapy would be limited at present. Decreasing the complexity of synergy testing methods, perhaps through automation[27] or the manufacturing of standardized synergy panels, could allow these methods to be adopted more widely in both research and, ultimately, clinical settings.

Maximizing the Usefulness of Synergy Data

In addition to simplifying synergy techniques, it will also be important to optimize the usefulness of the data generated by synergy testing. A great deal of information obtained from synergy studies, particularly time-kill assays and PK/PD models, is not used in traditional synergy definitions but may be of value in establishing clinical efficacy or optimal dosing regimens. For example, if bacterial killing after 6 hours of drug exposure is most predictive of clinical outcome for a certain drug, then an assay could be developed that specifically quantifies killing at 6 hours to simplify testing and improve predictive value. Similarly, data from PK/PD models could be used to optimize dose timing (eg, the administration of synergistic drugs to a patient simultaneously vs at staggered intervals) and to determine whether drugs with dose-dependent toxicities could be given at lower concentrations if used in combinations, thereby reducing side effects without sacrificing efficacy.

SUMMARY

The usefulness of combination antimicrobial therapy is evidenced by the ubiquity and efficacy of commonly used antibiotic combinations and by the recent introduction of broad-spectrum β-lactam–β-lactamase inhibitor combinations such as ceftazidime–avibactam and meropenem–vaborbactam, which can treat gram-negative bacteria that contain a *Klebsiella pneumoniae* carbapenemase enzyme, one of the most threatening antimicrobial resistance mechanisms known.[76] A host of literature describing combinations with in vitro activity against multidrug-resistant bacteria suggests that there are additional combination options within the armamentarium of existing antibiotics that may have usefulness in the treatment of patients infected with multidrug-resistant bacteria. More data, especially data that include the results of in vitro testing and clinical outcomes from the same bacterial isolates, as well as advances in synergy testing methods, are needed to determine which of these combinations will be most effective in combatting multidrug-resistant infections.

REFERENCES

1. Keshavjee S, Farmer PE. Tuberculosis, drug resistance, and the history of modern medicine. N Engl J Med 2012;367(10):931–6.
2. Hinshaw C, Feldman WH, Pfuetze KH. Treatment of tuberculosis with streptomycin; a summary of observations on one hundred cases. J Am Med Assoc 1946;132(13):778–82.
3. Daniel TM. The history of tuberculosis. Respir Med 2006;100(11):1862–70.
4. Crofton J, Mitchison DA. Streptomycin resistance in pulmonary tuberculosis. Br Med J 1948;11(2):1009–15.
5. World Health Organization. Guidelines for treatment of drug-susceptible tuberculosis and patient care, 2017 update. Geneva: World Health Organization; 2017. Available at: https://www.who.int/tb/publications/2017/dstb_guidance_2017/en/.
6. Mcgrath M, Gey van pittius NC, Van helden PD, et al. Mutation rate and the emergence of drug resistance in Mycobacterium tuberculosis. J Antimicrob Chemother 2014;69(2):292–302.
7. Gillespie SH. Evolution of drug resistance in Mycobacterium tuberculosis: clinical and molecular perspective. Antimicrob Agents Chemother 2002;46(2):267–74.
8. Rice LB. The Maxwell Finland lecture: for the duration– rational antibiotic administration in an era of antimicrobial resistance and Clostridium difficile. Clin Infect Dis 2008;46(4):491–6.
9. Tamma PD, Cosgrove SE, Maragakis LL. Combination therapy for treatment of infections with gram-negative bacteria. Clin Microbiol Rev 2012;25(3):450–70.
10. Eliopoulos GM, Eliopoulos CT. Antibiotic combinations: should they be tested? Clin Microbiol Rev 1988;1(2):139–56.
11. Bushby SRM. Trimethoprim-sulfamethoxazole: in vitro microbiological aspects. J Infect Dis 1973;128(Suppl):S442–62.
12. Hitchings GH. Mechanism of action of trimethoprim-sulfamethoxazole—I. J Infect Dis 1973;128(Suppl):S433–6.
13. Drawz SM, Bonomo RA. Three decades of β-lactamase inhibitors. Clin Microbiol Rev 2010;23(1):160–201.

14. Brennan-Krohn T, Pironti A, Kirby JE. Synergistic activity of colistin-containing combinations against colistin-resistant *Enterobacteriaceae*. Antimicrob Agents Chemother 2018. https://doi.org/10.1128/AAC.00873-18.
15. Moellering RC, Weinberg AN. Studies on antibiotic synergism against enterococci. II. Effect of various antibiotics on the uptake of 14 C-labeled streptomycin by enterococci. J Clin Invest 1971;50(12):2580–4.
16. Vaara M. Agents that increase the permeability of the outer membrane. Microbiol Rev 1992;56(3):395–411.
17. Phee LM, Betts JW, Bharathan B, et al. Colistin and fusidic acid, a novel potent synergistic combination for treatment of multidrug-resistant Acinetobacter baumannii infections. Antimicrob Agents Chemother 2015;59(8):4544–50.
18. Gavaldà J, Torres C, Tenorio C, et al. Efficacy of ampicillin plus ceftriaxone in treatment of experimental endocarditis due to Enterococcus faecalis strains highly resistant to aminoglycosides. Antimicrob Agents Chemother 1999;43(3): 639–46.
19. Mainardi JL, Gutmann L, Acar JF, et al. Synergistic effect of amoxicillin and cefotaxime against Enterococcus faecalis. Antimicrob Agents Chemother 1995;39(9): 1984–7. https://doi.org/10.1128/AAC.39.9.1984.
20. Baddour LM, Wilson WR, Bayer AS, et al. Infective endocarditis in adults: diagnosis, antimicrobial therapy, and management of complications. Circulation 2015;132(15):1435–86.
21. Zimmerli W, Sendi P. The role of rifampin against staphylococcal biofilm infections in vitro, in animal models, and in orthopedic device-related infections. Antimicrob Agents Chemother 2018;63(2). https://doi.org/10.1128/AAC.01746-18.
22. Goldstein BP. Resistance to rifampicin: a review. J Antibiot (Tokyo) 2014;67(9): 625–30.
23. Hirsch EB, Guo B, Chang KT, et al. Assessment of antimicrobial combinations for Klebsiella pneumoniae carbapenemase-producing K. pneumoniae. J Infect Dis 2013;207(5):786–93.
24. Louie A, Liu W, Vanguilder M, et al. Combination treatment with meropenem plus levofloxacin is synergistic against pseudomonas aeruginosa infection in a murine model of Pneumonia. J Infect Dis 2015;211(8):1326–33.
25. Descourouez JL, Jorgenson MR, Wergin JE, et al. Fosfomycin synergy in vitro with amoxicillin, daptomycin, and linezolid against vancomycin-resistant enterococcus faecium from renal transplant patients with infected urinary stents. Antimicrob Agents Chemother 2013;57(3):1518–20.
26. Toledo PVM, Aranha Junior AA, Arend LN, et al. Activity of antimicrobial combinations against KPC-2-Producing Klebsiella pneumoniae in a rat model and time-kill assay. Antimicrob Agents Chemother 2015;59(7):4301–4.
27. Brennan-Krohn T, Truelson KA, Smith KP, et al. Screening for synergistic activity of antimicrobial combinations against carbapenem-resistant Enterobacteriaceae using inkjet printer-based technology. J Antimicrob Chemother 2017;72(10): 2775–81.
28. Bergen PJ, Forrest A, Bulitta JB, et al. Clinically relevant plasma concentrations of colistin in combination with imipenem enhance pharmacodynamic activity against multidrug-resistant Pseudomonas aeruginosa at multiple inocula. Antimicrob Agents Chemother 2011;55(11):5134–42.
29. Sopirala MM, Mangino JE, Gebreyes WA, et al. Synergy testing by etest, microdilution checkerboard, and time-kill methods for pan-drug-resistant Acinetobacter baumannii. Antimicrob Agents Chemother 2010;54(11):4678–83.

30. Smith JR, Barber KE, Raut A, et al. β-Lactam combinations with daptomycin provide synergy against vancomycin-resistant Enterococcus faecalis and Enterococcus faecium. J Antimicrob Chemother 2014;70(6):1738–43.

31. Norden CW, Wentzel H, Keleti E. Comparison of techniques for measurement of in vitro antibiotic synergism. J Infect Dis 1979;140(4):629–33.

32. Bayer AS, Morrison JO. Disparity between timed-kill and checkerboard methods for determination of in vitro bactericidal interactions of vancomycin plus rifampin versus methicillin-susceptible and -resistant Staphylococcus aureus. Antimicrob Agents Chemother 1984;26(2):220–3.

33. White RL, Burgess DS, Manduru M, et al. Comparison of three different in vitro methods of detecting synergy: time-kill, checkerboard, and E test. Antimicrob Agents Chemother 1996;40(8):1914–8.

34. Ryan RW, Kwasnik I, Tilton RC. Methodological variation in antibiotic synergy tests against enterococci. J Clin Microbiol 1981;13(1):73–5.

35. Leber AL. Synergism testing: broth microdilution checkerboard and broth macrodilution methods. In: Leber AL, editor. Clinical microbiology procedures handbook. 4th edition. Washington, DC: ASM Press; 2016. p. 5.16.1–5.16.23.

36. CLSI. Performance standards for antimicrobial susceptibility testing. 29th edition. Wayne (PA): Clinical and Laboratory Standards Institute; 2019. CLSI Supplement M100.

37. Odds FC. Synergy, antagonism, and what the chequerboard puts between them. J Antimicrob Chemother 2003;52:1.

38. Clinical and Laboratory Standards Institute. M07: methods for dilution antimicrobial susceptibility tests for bacteria that grow aerobically. 11th edition. Wayne (PA): Clinical and Laboratory Standards Institute; 2018.

39. Greco WR, Bravo G, Parsons JC. The search for synergy: a critical review from a response surface perspective. Pharmacol Rev 1995;47(2):331–85.

40. Berenbaum MC. A method for testing for synergy with any number of agents. J Infect Dis 1978;137(2):122–30.

41. Berenbaum MC, Yu VL, Felegie TP. Synergy with double and triple antibiotic combinations compared. J Antimicrob Chemother 1983;12(6):555–63.

42. CLSI. Performance standards for antimicrobial disk susceptibility tests. 13th edition. Wayne (PA): Clinical and Laboratory Standards Institute; 2018. CLSI Standard M02.

43. Pillai SK, Moellering RC Jr, Eliopoulos GM. Antimicrobial combinations. In: Lorian V, editor. Antibiotics in laboratory medicine. Lippincott Williams & Wilkins; 2005. p. 365–440.

44. Stein C, Makarewicz O, Bohnert JA, et al. Three dimensional checkerboard synergy analysis of colistin, meropenem, tigecycline against multidrug-resistant clinical Klebsiella pneumonia isolates. PLoS One 2015;10(6). https://doi.org/10.1371/journal.pone.0126479.

45. Doern CD. When does 2 plus 2 equal 5? A review of antimicrobial synergy testing. J Clin Microbiol 2014;52(12):4124–8.

46. Leber AL. Etest. In: Leber A, editor. Clinical microbiology procedures handbook. 4th edition. Washington, DC: ASM Press; 2016. p. 5.3.

47. Pankey GA, Ashcraft DS, Dornelles A. Comparison of 3 Etest® methods and time-kill assay for determination of antimicrobial synergy against carbapenemase-producing Klebsiella species. Diagn Microbiol Infect Dis 2013; 77(3):220–6.

48. Leber AL. Time-kill assay for determining synergy. In: Leber AL, editor. Clinical microbiology procedures handbook. 4th edition. Washington, DC: ASM Press; 2016. p. 5.14.3.1–5.14.3.6.
49. Clinical and Laboratory Standards Institute (CLSI). Methods for determining bactericidal activity of antimicrobial agents; approved guideline. CLSI document M26-A. Wayne, PA: Clinical and Laboratory Standards Institute; 1999.
50. Drusano GL. Pre-clinical in vitro infection models. Curr Opin Pharmacol 2017;36: 100–6.
51. Blaser J. In-vitro model for simultaneous simulation of the serum kinetics of two drugs with different half-lives. J Antimicrob Chemother 1985;15(Suppl A):125–30.
52. Lenhard JR, Thamlikitkul V, Silveira FP, et al. Polymyxin-resistant, carbapenem-resistant Acinetobacter baumannii is eradicated by a triple combination of agents that lack individual activity. J Antimicrob Chemother 2017;72(5):1415–20.
53. Landersdorfer CB, Yadav R, Rogers KE, et al. Combating carbapenem-resistant Acinetobacter baumannii by an optimized imipenem-plus-Tobramycin dosage regimen: prospective validation via hollow-fiber infection and mathematical modeling. Antimicrob Agents Chemother 2018;62(4). https://doi.org/10.1128/AAC.02053-17.
54. Louie A, Heine HS, Kim K, et al. Use of an in vitro pharmacodynamic model to derive a linezolid regimen that optimizes bacterial kill and prevents emergence of resistance in Bacillus anthracis. Antimicrob Agents Chemother 2008;52(7): 2486–96.
55. Bulman ZP, Chen L, Walsh TJ, et al. Polymyxin combinations combat *Escherichia coli* harboring *mcr-1* and *bla$_{NDM-5}$*: preparation for a postantibiotic era. MBio 2017;8(4) [pii:e00540-17].
56. Marshall S, Hujer AM, Rojas LJ, et al. Can ceftazidime-avibactam and aztreonam overcome β-lactam resistance conferred by metallo-β-lactamases in Enterobacteriaceae? Antimicrob Agents Chemother 2017;61(4). https://doi.org/10.1128/AAC.02243-16.
57. Abdelraouf K, Kim A, Krause KM, et al. In vivo efficacy of plazomicin alone or in combination with meropenem or tigecycline against Enterobacteriaceae isolates exhibiting various resistance mechanisms in an immunocompetent murine septicemia model. Antimicrob Agents Chemother 2018;62(8). https://doi.org/10.1128/AAC.01074-18.
58. Andes D, Craig WA. Animal model pharmacokinetics and pharmacodynamics: a critical review. Int J Antimicrob Agents 2002;19(4):261–8.
59. Zuluaga AF, Salazar BE, Rodriguez CA, et al. Neutropenia induced in outbred mice by a simplified low-dose cyclophosphamide regimen: characterization and applicability to diverse experimental models of infectious diseases. BMC Infect Dis 2006;6(1):55.
60. Moellering RC, Weinberg AN. Studies on antibiotic synergism against enterococci. J Clin Invest 1971. https://doi.org/10.1172/JCI106758.
61. Chow JW. Aminoglycoside resistance in enterococci. Clin Infect Dis 2000;31(2): 586–9.
62. Doi Y, Chambers HF. Penicillins and β-lactamase inhibitors. In: Bennett JE, Dolin R, Blaser MJ, editors. Mandell, Douglas, and Bennett's principles and practice of infectious diseases, updated edition. 8th edition. Philadelphia: Saunders; 2015. p. 263–77.
63. Zinner SH, Mayer KH. Sulfonamides and trimethoprim. In: Bennett JE, Dolin R, Blaser MJ, editors. Mandell, Douglas, and Bennett's principles and practice of

infectious diseases, updated edition. 8th edition. Philadelphia: Saunders; 2015. p. 410–8.

64. Tängdén T, Hickman RA, Forsberg P, et al. Evaluation of double- and triple-antibiotic combinations for VIM- and NDM-producing klebsiella pneumoniae by in vitro time-kill experiments. Antimicrob Agents Chemother 2014;58(3):1757–62.

65. Lim TP, Cai Y, Hong Y, et al. In vitro pharmacodynamics of various antibiotics in combination against extensively drug-resistant Klebsiella pneumoniae. Antimicrob Agents Chemother 2015;59(5):2515–24.

66. Souli M, Rekatsina PD, Chryssouli Z, et al. Does the activity of the combination of imipenem and colistin in vitro exceed the problem of resistance in metallo-β-lactamase-producing Klebsiella pneumoniae isolates? Antimicrob Agents Chemother 2009;53(5):2133–5.

67. Bergen PJ, Bulman ZP, Saju S, et al. Polymyxin combinations: pharmacokinetics and pharmacodynamics for rationale use. Pharmacotherapy 2015;35(1):34–42.

68. Oliva A, Scorzolini L, Castaldi D, et al. Double-carbapenem regimen, alone or in combination with colistin, in the treatment of infections caused by carbapenem-resistant Klebsiella pneumoniae (CR-Kp). J Infect 2017;74(1):103–6.

69. Klastersky J, Cappel R, Daneau D. Clinical significance of in vitro synergism between antibiotics in gram-negative infections. Antimicrob Agents Chemother 1972;2(6):470–5.

70. de Maio Carrillho CMD, Gaudereto JJ, Martins RCR, et al. Colistin-resistant Enterobacteriaceae infections: clinical and molecular characterization and analysis of in vitro synergy. Diagn Microbiol Infect Dis 2017;87(3):253–7.

71. Daikos GL, Tsaousi S, Tzouvelekis LS, et al. Carbapenemase-producing Klebsiella pneumoniae bloodstream infections: lowering mortality by antibiotic combination schemes and the role of carbapenems. Antimicrob Agents Chemother 2014;58(4):2322–8.

72. Gutiérrez-Gutiérrez B, Salamanca E, de Cueto M, et al. Effect of appropriate combination therapy on mortality of patients with bloodstream infections due to carbapenemase-producing Enterobacteriaceae (INCREMENT): a retrospective cohort study. Lancet Infect Dis 2017;17(7):726–34.

73. Aaron SD, Vandemheen KL, Ferris W, et al. Combination antibiotic susceptibility testing to treat exacerbations of cystic fibrosis associated with multiresistant bacteria: a randomised, double-blind, controlled clinical trial. Lancet 2005;366: 463–71.

74. Aaron SD. Antibiotic synergy testing should not be routine for patients with cystic fibrosis who are infected with multiresistant bacterial organisms. Paediatr Respir Rev 2007;8(3):256–61.

75. Saiman L. Clinical utility of synergy testing for multidrug-resistant Pseudomonas aeruginosa isolated from patients with cystic fibrosis: "the motion for. Paediatr Respir Rev 2007;8(3):249–55.

76. Ramos-Castañeda JA, Ruano-Ravina A, Barbosa-Lorenzo R, et al. Mortality due to KPC carbapenemase-producing Klebsiella pneumoniae infections: systematic review and meta-analysis: mortality due to KPC Klebsiella pneumoniae infections. J Infect 2018;76(5):438–48.

Clinical Microbiology in Underresourced Settings

Ellen Jo Baron, PhD

KEYWORDS

- Diagnostic bacteriology • Challenges • Personnel • Infrastructure • Supplies
- Governmental support

KEY POINTS

- Diagnostic services for the major diseases of underresourced settings, including human immunodeficiency virus, malaria, tuberculosis, and hepatitis, are often performed in donor-supported or government reference laboratories, not necessarily connected with basic bacteriology laboratories nor with each other, leading to duplication of efforts, inefficiency, and lack of integrated health care services.
- Although noncommunicable diseases (mainly cardiovascular, cancer, metabolic) account for greater than 70% of deaths in low and middle income countries, lower respiratory tract infections and diarrhea are the 2 major causes of death among communicable diseases. No generalized statistics are available on the death toll due to sepsis, bacterial meningitis, bacterial pneumonia, and other infections.
- Timely results from culture-based clinical microbiology and manual antimicrobial susceptibility testing can lead to improvement in patient outcomes, early detection of emerging infectious disease or resistance trends, better institutional infection control, and early detection of biothreat agent deployment.
- Challenges to building basic microbiology capacity in underresourced settings fall within the realms of personnel and management, supplies and reagents, infrastructure, and the policies and attitudes at every level of leadership within the health care system and the government.
- With perseverance, patience, and a long-term perspective, sustainable diagnostic microbiology services can be developed.

The global Sustainable Development Goals adopted by the United Nations in 2015, with the expectation of fulfillment by 2030, include 1 health care–related goal: "Good Health and Wellbeing."[1] An integral component of good health is freedom from disease. In underresourced settings, the burden of infectious diseases is higher than in resource-rich environments.[2] The World Bank reports that 73% of the 189 listed countries are considered to be middle or lower income, with annual income

Disclosure Statement: The author has nothing to disclose.
Stanford University School of Medicine, Stanford, CA, USA
E-mail address: ejbaron@stanford.edu

less than $4000. More than three-quarters of the world's population live in low and middle income countries (LMICs).[3] Most LMICs should be considered as underresourced settings, and they are primarily located in sub-Saharan Africa, India, and Southeast Asia. Although noncommunicable diseases (eg, cardiovascular, cancer, diabetes) account for greater than 70% of all deaths, communicable diseases still kill millions annually. According to the World Health Organization (WHO), lower respiratory tract infections and diarrheal disease account for most deaths caused by communicable diseases worldwide, with communicable (nontuberculosis) lower respiratory tract infections killing greater than 3 million people and diarrheal disease accounting for greater than 1 million deaths in 2016.[4,5]

The major individual infectious diseases for which statistics are available include human immunodeficiency virus (HIV), malaria, tuberculosis, and hepatitis. Modern molecular or rapid antigen tests are available and often supplied at low cost to high-burden developing countries (as defined by the World Health Organization). Laboratory testing for these major diseases is often performed at reference laboratories under government-supported or donor-supported programs. One problem with these programs is their lack of integration. Funding and patient management are done in silos, with little or no coordination. Thus, laboratories that perform molecular testing for tuberculosis may be using the same platform as those performing hepatitis or HIV tests, but they are located in different buildings or rooms and they do not share equipment. Personnel trained to perform rapid antigen tests for malaria are not trained or paid to do any other testing on patients who present with febrile disease, despite that they may have Ebola or typhoid, common in the same settings. This is among the many challenges of establishing diagnostic microbiology services in low-resource settings. Because major international efforts are already directed toward detection and eradication of HIV, malaria, tuberculosis, and hepatitis, albeit in independently organized and executed programs, this article focuses on the author's experience in developing basic culture-centered microbiology laboratory diagnostic capability for the common bacterial diseases affecting patients in underresourced settings.

Neglected tropical diseases, including such esoteric diseases as yaws, Buruli ulcer, Chagas disease, leishmaniasis, leprosy, schistosomiasis, onchocerciasis, deep mycoses, and (currently more common) dengue, are also monitored. However, patients in underresourced settings often suffer from bacterial pneumonia, urinary tract infections, bacteremia and sepsis, wound infections, bacterial or cryptococcal meningitis, and bacterial diarrhea, for which there are no specific global statistics. A definitive diagnosis for any of the latter diseases can be determined with relatively simple laboratory tests within the realm of basic microbiology. Knowing the etiologic agent and its antimicrobial profile allows targeted and effective therapy.

A diagnostic microbiology laboratory adds value to a health care system and overall population wellbeing in at least 5 areas:

- Individual case management by detection and identification of microbial agents of bloodstream infections, pneumonia, wound infections, meningitis, diarrhea, and urinary tract infections
- Detection of emerging antibiotic resistance and prevention of spread of resistance
- Hospital infection control
- Early detection of microbial pathogens with public health importance, including potential biothreat agents
- Support of outbreak investigations.

However, primarily, the initial premise for performing diagnostic microbiology tests, including antimicrobial susceptibilities (ASTs) when warranted, is that the treating health care provider will use that information to enhance the individual patient's management with the expectation of an improved outcome. Years of studies looking at the benefit of timely microbiological information support this principle.[6–9] Microbiologists in appropriately resourced settings base their practice (and their careers) on the timely provision of results to clinicians or others who need that information for patient management. In some environments, empiric treatment decisions have already been made and the impact of the results delivery is less dramatic (and greeted with less enthusiasm). Nevertheless, occasional unexpected findings often lead to improved patient outcomes, deescalation of certain antibiotics, and overall better health.

An attempt to establish or improve clinical microbiology practices is based on the belief that the laboratory results will be valued and used. This is an assumption that may not always be correct. It seems that there are 2 types of underresourced settings for clinical microbiology.

Setting 1: Physicians acknowledge that it is possible for a microbiology laboratory to deliver useful diagnostic test results that will enable them to more expediently or correctly manage the infectious diseases presented by their patients. Either the caregivers had some training in this discipline in medical school or postdoctoral studies, or they witnessed improved patient outcomes based on data-driven interventions or they heard about it from another source, such as a respected colleague or even a television program. In such a setting, there is some incentive for improved microbiology services, and the process of developing such a system is easier.

Setting 2: The value of accurate diagnostic microbiology test results has not been demonstrated. In some cases, there were microbiology laboratories that had not delivered results that were correct or not in time for any intervention based on those results. In other cases, there were no diagnostic microbiology laboratories so caregivers had never learned to request laboratory tests or include such test results in their patient management activities. In such a setting, the road to sustainable high-quality microbiology services is longer and bumpier.

In addition to the reception (by the physician or caregiver) given to microbiology laboratory results (positive, grateful, interested, or bothered, indifferent), there is the added challenge of training the laboratory workers in accepted practices to assure accurate and timely results. The success of those training endeavors depends on the laboratory environment in the region. Laboratory workers in underresourced settings may be well-trained in didactic microbiology but have little hands-on experience, or they may have very little microbiology knowledge at all. The success of capacity-building efforts depends on the motivation of the laboratory workers to learn new techniques, dedication to their job, pride in their profession, and other intangible aspects that are taken for granted in more developed health care environments. It should be recognized that having strong and clear communication between trainers and laboratory workers is essential, and language differences are major barriers that must be surmounted. Even if an expert uses a translator with good general bilingual capability, if the translator does not also have background knowledge or expertise in microbiology, concepts and practices may not be clearly communicated. At least 1 aspect of microbiology helps to overcome this obstacle: the visual and interactive nature of basic manual microbiology, in which correct practices can be modeled and practiced under direct observation. The author spent a month working side-by-side with a microbiologist in a referral hospital in Nepal with neither of us understanding the language of the other; however, we learned together and much microbiology knowledge was shared.

Another challenge in resource-poor environments is developing the infrastructure needed for good laboratory practices. In fact, a donor will often assist with construction of facilities and providing initial instrumentation. Although sourcing and purchasing equipment and supplies should be easy (given external support), many donors do not include the cost of maintenance or provision of ongoing quality control (QC) materials, and both of those essential activities are often neglected. The result is that equipment fails to function over time and eventually is not useable. Lack of QC practices results in test results that are incorrect, with the predictable outcome of lack of trust among ordering caregivers; decreasing numbers of test orders; and, finally, lack of practice and further degradation of skills among the laboratory workers: a downward spiral.

For all of these reasons, developing laboratory capacity in resource-constrained settings requires a long-term commitment from those doing the training and support; immense patience; and, ultimately, a change in culture within the entire health care setting. Depending on the health care sector (private vs government or public) the role of leadership at every level cannot be overestimated.

EXAMPLES OF PERSONNEL ISSUES

In a few countries in which the author has worked (**Fig. 1**), the percent of laboratory workers versus the total population varied dramatically (based on 2010 WHO Laboratory Workforce data).[10]

Numbers do not tell the whole story, however. Education and national priorities also play a strong role in the level of microbiology laboratory support available in a country, particularly in the public sector. Over the past few years, for example, there has been a strong emphasis to improve laboratory services in many African countries supported by the African Society for Laboratory Medicine (ASLM.org). Using a program called Stepwise Laboratory Quality Improvement Process Towards Accreditation (SLIPTA), the WHO Regional Office for Africa established a program to improve quality of public health laboratories to the 15189 standard of the International Organization for Standardization (ISO). In 2014, greater than 80% of South African laboratories were accredited, but only 15% of laboratories in other African countries were accredited.[11] Since then, 62 additional laboratories, many in Ethiopia, Kenya, Zambia, and South

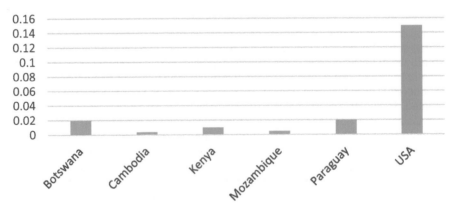

Fig. 1. Percent of population working in medical laboratories in selected underresourced countries based on 2010 data.

Africa, have become accredited to another standard: Strengthening Laboratory Management Toward Accreditation (SLMTA), a structured quality improvement program that concentrates on laboratory quality management systems in resource-limited settings.[12] The pan-African laboratory organization holds annual meetings, supports courses and workshops, and fosters a sense of professionalism and pride in laboratory workers, encouraging laboratory personnel to strive for the recognition that achieving an accepted quality standard affords. Several laboratories in Vietnam and the Caribbean region also have used the SLMTA method and become accredited. Only 1 laboratory in Cambodia (nearest neighbor to Vietnam), for example, is ISO accredited and only since December of 2018.[13] In contrast, 31 laboratories in Paraguay, a country with less than one-third the population of Cambodia, have achieved that level.[14] These statistics underscore the variation seen in attitude toward quality laboratories and thus the degree of difficulty in establishing strong laboratory services in LMICs. Each situation is unique.

Although not all personnel in challenging low-resource environments lack motivation or enthusiasm for improving microbiological skills, those interested and dedicated individuals are the minority in public laboratories. A key problem is that the government wages are not sufficient to support a family, or even a single person who is not living at home with parents. Additional income can be generated by doing sanctioned workshops and day-trips to other laboratories for assessment purposes or other reasons. The worker is paid a per diem for the travel, but the money is saved and the worker stays with friends or family and does not use the per diem for expenses. Enterprising microbiologists can create their own private laboratories and siphon off excess supplies from the government laboratory to cut down on expenses. In some cases, samples that arrive in the public laboratory can be taken to the private laboratory for testing, and the payment for the test then goes into the private laboratory profits. In some settings, government laboratories accept specimens from private reference laboratories or individuals for testing, and the revenue is shared among the workers. Rather than serving as a public service laboratory, as does the Centers for Disease Control in Atlanta, Georgia, the public laboratories in these countries are in competition with private laboratories, and, in some cases, they provide kickback payments to physicians or laboratory owners for each sample received. Note that, in these types of settings, it is very rare for patients to have any insurance coverage so that all testing costs are out of pocket. In fact, the reluctance to have laboratory tests performed due to the cost is a major barrier to general good health in these countries. An excellent study by Pai and colleagues[15] highlighted the circuitous route that many tuberculosis patients in India took before finally receiving the correct diagnosis and being placed on correct therapy. The private (often not accredited) health care provider system within LMICs is the first stop for many patients based on the perception of lowest cost (not always true and certainly not true over the course of many visits).

Despite low wages, jobs in public laboratories are sought out in at least 1 low-resource country and this is probably the case in others. Why? Public laboratory workers are hired for life. They cannot be fired or laid-off and, when they reach retirement age, they receive a pension. Their wages are not ever reduced for poor performance (or even no performance); however, they are never rewarded with bonuses or other than generic incremental pay increases. There is no incentive to show up on time, show initiative, or work harder. And there is no sanction for not staying at work all day, for taking long lunch hours, or making errors. And the manager is often in the same situation and feels that there is nothing to be done to stimulate employees to do better work.

Education, especially basic microbiology (both didactic and laboratory-based), is a key differentiator among resource-poor countries. In some Central American and South American countries, laboratory technology is a respected field and microbiology is an essential component of the curriculum. Graduates of the technical programs are proud to be microbiologists and acknowledge that its practice requires more judgment than some other laboratory disciplines that are more automated. This is becoming more common in many sub-Saharan African countries as well. However, access to good teaching materials, teachers with scientific backgrounds or practical experience, and books in the language of the country are lacking in some low-resource settings in India and Southeast Asia.

In general, cultural differences are also a challenge in some LMICs. The altruistic goal of communicating a key laboratory finding to a physician that saves a patient's life or limb does not seem to be present in many workers. Perhaps because the physicians have not been accustomed to using timely data for patient management decisions, they have not rewarded microbiologists when good information was received. The timeworn exhortation often used in my training, "What if that spinal fluid was from your mother?," to spur rapid action does not seem to hold the same importance in some low-resource settings. Laboratory workers tend to rely totally on their standard operating procedures (SOPs), if there are some. Being creative or making a decision about how to manage a culture result that has not been specifically addressed in the SOPs is rare. One example is a blood culture isolate that could not be identified using the reagents available. It was a gram-positive coccus in chains, catalase-negative but not a known type of streptococcus. The laboratory thus was unable to perform ASTs because the document used for interpreting AST results did not have a category for this organism. In more advanced laboratories, technologists would be expected to choose the closest category to use for interpretive results and write a comment to that effect on the report. This type of creative problem-solving must be nurtured and developed in some settings.

A recent paper from the Bacteriology in Low Resource Settings working group outlines a framework for implementation of clinical microbiology services in low-resource settings.[16] The group advocates for conventional culture techniques until the high-technology diagnostics now used in most resource-rich locations become more easily obtainable and adaptable to the low-resource setting. The group also advocated for prioritizing the types of specimens cultured, with blood cultures being the most important. Performing quality blood cultures, however, has its own set of challenges, and many laboratories in LMICs do not perform blood cultures at all. Commercial blood culture media bottles are expensive; many are made for instruments that the laboratories cannot afford or that have stopped working due to lack of maintenance. Homemade blood culture bottles require difficult-to-obtain reagents, such as sodium polyanethol sulfonate, and a source of glass bottles and stoppers. In that laboratory in Nepal mentioned previously, we used small discarded whiskey bottles (collected from a nearby bar) and cotton stoppers: not an ideal solution. Another problem with blood cultures in LMICs is the reluctance of health care workers to obtain enough blood for a reliable result. Realize how difficult it is now in developed locations to obtain 2 separate blood cultures with 10 mL blood in each bottle and multiply that difficulty by at least 5 times. Patients feel that they are losing too much precious blood and they object strenuously, so many blood cultures in LMIC settings consist of 1 bottle. Additionally, it may be difficult to thoroughly disinfect the phlebotomy site due to lack of washing (maybe lack of clean water) and years of accumulated dirt on the skin; therefore, contamination by *Bacillus* species or staphylococci is more common than in developed countries. Chlorhexidine is too expensive, so povidone iodine (Betadine) is the most common disinfectant, and it can become contaminated with hardy environmental organisms. A recent publication undertaken by workers in the Fund for Innovative New Diagnostics (FIND) outlines the difficulties of implementing blood cultures in resource-limited settings, and suggests a product profile to overcome some of those issues.[17]

However, although the infrastructure and consumables challenges are listed in the FIND publication, and are potentially solvable, the cultural change that must occur at the leadership level and at the individual worker level are not mentioned and deserve consideration. In addition, although blood cultures may be the most important first challenge, the other infectious disease specimen types must be managed to develop full-service microbiology in these settings. Perhaps a more realistic view of the current situation is presented in a recent series on pathology laboratory services in LMICs.[18] The investigators found 4 major barriers to optimal laboratory performance: lack of human resources or workforce capacity (to which the author adds lack of workforce incentives); inadequate education and training; infrastructure issues (which can be solved); and insufficient quality management, including working to achieve standards and, ultimately, accreditation. Note that laboratory personnel must want accreditation and the staff must believe in the goal enough to do all the work needed to get there. These concepts are not to be taken for granted in low-resource settings.

EXAMPLES OF SUPPLIES ISSUES

In many countries, government laboratories cannot simply order the reagents or supplies that they need when they need them. In 1 African country, for example, supplies could be ordered only once a year, in September, and the shipments began to arrive in March. It is impossible to predict the volume of work more than a year in advance, and so the laboratories routinely ran out of supplies before the next year arrived. When there were no supplies, testing stopped. In addition to limits on timing of orders, only the reagents listed on the national supply list could be ordered. In the absence of a supply list, laboratories would order items but would not receive the same item or, most often, they would receive an item from a different manufacturer, often of lower quality. The government supply office would be tasked with cutting expenditures, and they could do this by purchasing inferior products at lower cost. Because no one in the supply office had any knowledge about laboratory procedures or the need for certain quality-controlled items, they had no problem with making substitutions as they saw fit. For example, if powder-free gloves were ordered, the gloves received would usually be powdered-gloves for physical examinations, which could be purchased in bulk for use in all health care settings. Gram stain reagents were another difficult item to keep in stock. The supply office could not imagine that a laboratory used so many Gram stain supplies, so they refused to send sufficient stock to last the entire period.

More expensive reagents, such as biochemical organism identification strips, were usually purchased with donor funds or donated outright. If purchased under a government purchase plan, dated reagents were often received very near the expiration date. Was it cheaper for the supply office or did someone in control receive a kickback for accepting such short-dated reagents? Due to their scarcity, such strips were used sparingly, and they would often expire. However, given their precious nature, they would continue to be used as long as possible, potentially delivering incorrect results, which would not be questioned but reported as such.

Many microbiology laboratories in low-resource settings cannot afford to purchase premade media and attempt to make their own. There are at least 2 major problems with this strategy. First, much of clinical microbiology initial organism identification depends on morphology and hemolysis on sheep (or horse) blood agar. However, horses are too expensive or too scarce in many low-resource areas, and wool sheep, at least, are not suitable for the climate. Thus the laboratories rely on human blood, either their own workers' blood or outdated blood bank blood, to make their blood and chocolate agar plates. Problems with human blood include antibodies to common pathogens and different hemolytic reactions, making recognition of common pathogens difficult or impossible.[19] The second problem with homemade media is the lack of QC practices or disregard of poor QC results. The use of specific organisms for routine QC requires a good storage system; ideally, a low temperature freezer, which is beyond the reach of most low-resource laboratories. Also, often, the technicians have made a small quantity of media just in time to use as their previous supply runs out, using valuable resources and taking time from actual microbiology culture interpretation. If the new media fails to pass QC, there is no option but to use it anyway. And the results of testing do not reflect this QC failure. For example, a batch of chocolate agar (Thayer-Martin agar was too difficult or expensive to attempt) failed to grow the QC *Neisseria gonorrhoeae* after 48 hours of incubation; however, given that there was no other supply, the laboratory plated patient genital samples onto this batch and reported out "no *N gonorrhoeae* isolated" without further comment. This sort of activity is partly due to a culture that does not nurture problem-solving or thinking outside the box so that the technicians do not readily appreciate the problem with their approach.

Transport media are another challenge. Standard swabs with transport media in sponges or ampoules are usually too expensive and laboratories may make their own transport systems. These homemade devices might even include homemade cotton swabs, which are not conducive to the survival of some fastidious pathogens. Just moving caregivers away from swabs for all specimens, including fluids and tissues, will be a daunting task but worth the effort. Trying to assure that urine specimens are kept cold after collection is another of the issues that plague microbiology laboratories in underresourced areas. Commercial cold packs are expensive, thus reused until they no longer function, and frozen plastic water bottles cannot stay frozen long enough.

RISING TO THE CHALLENGE

Despite the relatively discouraging environment for clinical bacteriology in some underresourced settings, improvements can always be made and some successes are possible. A dedicated and motivating leader, even at the microbiology laboratory supervisor level, can set a high standard and the staff will rise to his or her expectations. Occasional technologists or technicians will be enthusiastic about learning new skills and will work hard to improve. For some, their objective is to be able to teach the subject in a local university or to start their own private laboratory, and those goals should be encouraged because any reason for performing better microbiology and extending better service to the community is a benefit. However, the outside expert or organization whose goal is microbiology laboratory capacity building must be prepared to dedicate many years to the project and to surmount many challenges. It is a source of pride to see the supervisor who has been nurtured for several years rise to a level of success that entails promotion to a higher position in that laboratory or in another laboratory, but then the task of mentoring the next supervisor must begin anew. Over years of working in underresourced settings, the author has developed several factors to consider for those who wish to help move microbiology to a higher standard in those settings.

Importance of Initial Assessment

What are the microbiology technologists doing now? A new outside advisor should plan to spend at least several weeks observing current workflow, work habits, techniques, and overall environment before ever attempting any interventions. Besides getting to know the system, this allows the laboratory staff to become familiar with the expert, develop some rapport, and lessen their initial suspicion. It also shows that the expert is not a drop-in and drop-out person who will spend minimal time and then leave without making any substantial contributions. It is important to assess the level of training that the workers have, which may be different among the staff members. What sorts of practices are they doing that are clearly incorrect and will need to be unlearned? How do they work together? Does everyone seem to ask a particular person questions about activities or protocols? Who is in charge (it may not be the boss of record)? What are the priorities of the staff? Does their family life take precedence over laboratory tasks? Who seems to be the most dedicated worker?

Importance of Infrastructure

What equipment, stocks, and supplies are available? Do workers perform appropriate equipment maintenance? Is the equipment functional? What about QC? Do they have QC reagents and are they being used correctly? In 1 laboratory, I discovered that the biological indicator ampoules used to monitor the autoclave function were being incubated but the ampoules were never broken to allow the media to mix with the spores. Nevertheless, they were all reported out as "passed QC." So not only was the test not done correctly, the result was not interpreted or reported correctly either. Having good microscopes is essential to good microbiology. Advisors usually need to adjust the microscopes, show the users how to clean the lenses, and to not remove glass slides from the stage when the oil lens is down.

How are results reported? Is there a computerized system? Do physicians have access to it? Does the system allow all the report comments necessary? Can the caregivers be called with critical results? Sometimes a lot of outside expertise is needed to improve an existing system or even to create it if none exists.

Utilization of Standard Operating Procedures and Other Written Materials

Not only should SOPs be available, but they must be adapted to the specific laboratory practice and understandable to the users. This usually entails having a set of procedures in the local language. Workers need to know where the SOPs are located and should have a very low threshold to check the SOPs when procedural questions arise. Emphasizing continued use of SOPs and teaching tools, laboratory job aids, and other work-simplifying tools is a constant task for the outside mentor. As stated by the Bacteriology in Low Resource Settings working group, site-appropriate and locally validated protocols and job aids are key components of quality improvement.[16] Note that outside experts often like to impose their own practice or ideas on the laboratory in which they are working, and those ideas or standards may not coincide totally with the local SOPs. This is a recipe for trouble because when the outside expert is gone, the laboratory is now without the knowledge-base that allowed those different protocols to function, and it is confusing and difficult to return to the original local SOPs. Outside mentors must be prepared to follow only the local SOPs, despite having more knowledge and wishing that they could go further (with an identification or to test another antibiotic). This can be frustrating, but it is in the best interests of sustainability.

Working Within the Local, Regional, and National Health Care System

Learn the local hierarchy, from the laboratory to the hospital management to the public health officers, in the area. Visit all the leaders in these areas before starting a project and continue to have regular meetings to discuss progress or ask for help with barriers. If the leadership is indifferent or hostile, the success of any endeavor is compromised. Microbiology must be conducted in concert with appropriate physician test requesting, good specimen collection and transport, and constant communication with physicians and pharmacists. Visiting experts need to coach the local laboratory microbiologists to work with nurses and physicians on proper test ordering and specimen collection. Sample collection guides should be created and disseminated, and then reinforced constantly. Laboratories should know what antibiotics are available in their setting and report AST results hierarchically based on local practice. Fostering pride in the profession and gaining the benefits of communication among peers is another goal to which an outside organization should aspire. Once the local microbiologists or other laboratory scientists begin to recognize their worth and the value of networking, they should be encouraged to get together for workshops, training, and sharing of advice and expertise. Having social media chat groups consisting of likeminded laboratorians will help develop the system and generalize good practices.

Being Patient

No change occurs quickly; this is true in the resource-rich laboratory environment but even truer in resource-limited settings. The outside mentors must be prepared to reteach the same lessons innumerable times, to remind workers to perform QC on a daily basis, and to sit quietly without interjecting their own ideas to allow technologists time to assess a culture and perform the appropriate follow-up testing. It is tempting to do the work yourself, to come in on weekends to check important cultures even when the official laboratory staff is enjoying a long 4-day holiday; however, that behavior by the mentor will not lead to sustainable change in local practice. The author has found that with a relatively motivated leader and a few enthusiastic staff working in a basic microbiology laboratory that did not previously exist and where the workers had virtually no specific training, the laboratory could function at a consistently acceptable level of quality after 2 years of continuous mentorship. The provision of correct culture results over this time period encourages physicians to order more tests, and the increasing numbers of specimens allows the laboratory workers to develop higher skills and gain experience. In return, the physicians' level of trust and reliance on the microbiology results contributes to a positive feedback loop.

SUMMARY

Basic diagnostic microbiology can be performed in underresourced settings without the use of any molecular or automated instruments. Even simple cultures and manual ASTs will save lives; prevent chronic disability; detect antimicrobial resistance; and, with good communication, inform the relevant authorities of emerging infectious disease trends. Although the challenges and barriers are formidable, the mentor will meet and work with wonderful people as students and collaborators. The ability to mentor the next generation of laboratory professionals, to reinforce idealism when it is discovered, and to use one's own skills and ideas that had remained dormant in the laboratory environment of the resource-rich setting is an opportunity that should be considered by the microbiologist with a suitable background and temperament.

REFERENCES

1. Sustainable development knowledge platform. Available at: https://sustainabledevelopment.un.org/. Accessed January 6, 2019.
2. Lozano R, Fullman N, Abate D, et al. Measuring progress from 1990 to 2017 and projecting attainment to 2030 of the health-related Sustainable Development Goals for 195 countries and territories: a systematic analysis for the Global Burden of Disease Study 2017. Lancet 2018;392(10159):2091–138.
3. WDI - the world by income and region. Available at: http://datatopics.worldbank.org/world-development-indicators/the-world-by-income-and-region.html. Accessed January 6, 2019.
4. Roser M, Ritchie H. Causes of death. Our World in data. 2018. Available at: https://ourworldindata.org/causes-of-death. Accessed January 6, 2019.
5. The top 10 causes of death. Available at: https://www.who.int/news-room/fact-sheets/detail/the-top-10-causes-of-death. Accessed January 6, 2019.
6. Reller LB, Weinstein MP, Peterson LR, et al. Role of clinical microbiology laboratories in the management and control of infectious diseases and the delivery of health care. Clin Infect Dis 2001;32(4):605–10.
7. Nguyen DT, Yeh E, Perry S, et al. Real-time PCR testing for *mecA* Reduces vancomycin usage and length of hospitalization for patients infected with methicillin-sensitive staphylococci. J Clin Microbiol 2010;48(3):785–90.
8. Galar A, Leiva J, Espinosa M, et al. Clinical and economic evaluation of the impact of rapid microbiological diagnostic testing. J Infect 2012;65(4):302–9.
9. Cattoir L, Coorevits L, Leroux-Roels I, et al. Improving timelines in reporting results from positive blood cultures: simulation of impact of rapid identification on therapy on a real-life cohort. Eur J Clin Microbiol Infect Dis 2018;37:2253–60.
10. World Health Organization. Global health workforce statistics – 2018 update. Geneva (Switzeland): Health Workforce; 2017. Available at: https://www.who.int/hrh/statistics/hwfstats/en/ http://who.int/hrh/statistics.
11. Schroeder LF, Amukele T. Medical laboratories in sub-Saharan Africa that meet international quality standards. Am J Clin Pathol 2014;141(6):791–5.
12. SLMTA | Strengthening laboratory management toward accreditation. Available at: https://slmta.org/accredited-labs/. Accessed January 6, 2019.
13. Vichea P. Cambodian lab first to receive quality award. Phnom Penh Post. 2018. Available at: https://www.phnompenhpost.com/national/cambodian-lab-first-receive-quality-award. Accessed January 6, 2019.
14. Laboratorios de ensayos | Conacyt. Available at: http://www.conacyt.gov.py/laboratorios-de-ensayos. Accessed January 6, 2019.
15. Yellapa V, Devadasan N, Krumeich A, et al. How patients navigate the diagnostic ecosystem in a fragmented health system: a qualitative study from India. Glob Health Action 2017;10(1):1350452.
16. Ombelet S, Ronat J-B, Walsh T, et al. Clinical bacteriology in low-resource settings: today's solutions. Lancet Infect Dis 2018;18(8):e248–58.
17. Dailey P, Osborn J, Ashley E, et al. Defining system requirements for simplified blood culture to enable widespread use in resource-limited settings. Diagnostics (Basel) 2019;9(1):10.
18. Wilson ML, Fleming KA, Kuti MA, et al. Access to pathology and laboratory medicine services: a crucial gap. Lancet 2018;391(10133):1927–38.
19. Yeh E, Pinsky BA, Banaei N, et al. Hair sheep blood, citrated or defibrinated, fulfills all requirements of blood agar for diagnostic microbiology laboratory tests. PLoS One 2009;4(7):e6141.

REFERENCES

Total Laboratory Automation

What Is Gained, What Is Lost, and Who Can Afford It?

Richard B. Thomson Jr, PhD, D(ABMM)[a,b,]*,
Erin McElvania, PhD, D(ABMM)[a]

KEYWORDS

- Microbiology automation • Microbiology cost savings • Microbiology efficiency
- Microbiology quality • Copan WASPLab • BD Kiestra TLA

KEY POINTS

- Microbiology laboratory automation is the greatest single change in clinical microbiology in decades.
- Automation reduces costs, improves quality, and shortens turnaround times.
- Automation changes the skill set needed by microbiology technologists.
- As laboratory test reimbursement continues to change from fee-for-service to value-based models, microbiology automation may provide a competitive advantage.

There have been many transformative moments in the history of clinical microbiology. For example, when Hans Christian Gram first added crystal violet and iodine to lung tissue, and looked into the microscope to see gram-positive cocci and gram-negative bacilli later identified as *Streptococcus pneumoniae* and *Klebsiella pneumonia*; when Robert Koch flashed a smile at his wife while explaining that the agar she recommended as a hardening agent worked great with bacterial culture media; or when Bauer and Kirby realized that the zones of inhibition around antimicrobial-containing disks predicted drug susceptibility. These are iconic examples of transformative moments in clinical microbiology. Early steps to fully automate the bacteriology portion of clinical microbiology laboratories is just such a moment. A laboratory occupying less space, with fewer technologists, dramatic improvements in efficiency, more

Disclosure Statement: Doctors R.B. Thomson and E. McElvania have received research funding and speaking honoraria from BD Kiestra in the past year.
[a] Department of Pathology and Laboratory Medicine, NorthShore University Health System, 2650 Ridge Avenue, Evanston, IL 60201, USA; [b] Department of Pathology and Laboratory Medicine, The University of Chicago Pritzker School of Medicine, Chicago, IL 60637, USA
* Corresponding author. Department of Pathology and Laboratory Medicine, NorthShore University Health System, 2650 Ridge Avenue, Evanston, IL 60045.
E-mail address: RThomson@northshore.org

Clin Lab Med 39 (2019) 371–389
https://doi.org/10.1016/j.cll.2019.05.002
0272-2712/19/© 2019 Elsevier Inc. All rights reserved.

accurate results, and reduced turnaround times (TAT) to important results are achievable now with full automation. This is a paradigm shift in clinical microbiology, representing the beginning of the future.[1-4]

Adopting laboratory automation is one of the greatest changes and challenges to our generation of clinical microbiologists. This article summarizes a review of the literature and personal opinion based on exposure to the two dominant automation systems available: BD Kiestra Total Laboratory Automation (TLA; Becton-Dickinson, Sparks, MD) and Copan WASPLab (Copan Diagnostics Inc, Murrieta, CA). Both offer "jaw dropping" innovations that change the profession. Software and hardware upgrades are occurring so frequently that any written side-by-side comparison is soon outdated. We explain how automation changes the laboratory, what is gained, what is lost, and whether one can afford to pay for automation. In total, the question becomes, can one afford not to automate?

AUTOMATED SYSTEMS: DEFINITIONS AND DIFFERENCES

Although there has been automation in other areas of microbiology, most notably automated blood culture incubation, automated antimicrobial susceptibility testing, and polymerase chain reaction testing, the backbone of laboratory effort continues to involve receiving clinical specimens, manually preparing smears, inoculating and streaking agar plates, loading incubators, unloading incubators, interpreting plates, performing identification and antimicrobial tests, reloading incubators, and repeating this process one or more times before discarding all plates and submitting a final report. Although the future will include automation in mycology, mycobacteriology, parasitology and automated integration of instrumentation listed previously, total laboratory automation in this review is defined as instrumentation that automates the bacteriology processes from specimen receiving to discarding plates.

There are two commercially available microbiology laboratory automation systems in the United States at this time: Kiestra (Becton Dickinson) and WASPLab (Copan Diagnostics Inc).[1,5] Each of the systems is modular and customizable for the size and needs of a laboratory and can consist of a front-end processing unit alone or with add-ons providing more complete automation. For purposes of this review, the three most common configuration-types to be installed are front-end processing, which we refer to as automated plating (**Fig. 1**); front-end processing plus automated incubation and plate imaging with plate delivery to a central plate retrieval area referred to as

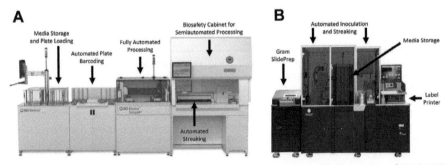

Fig. 1. (*A*) Illustration of Kiestra InoculA automated plating system. (*B*) Illustration of WASP-DT automated plating system. (*Courtesy of* [A] Becton Dickinson, Sparks, MD; and [B] Copan Diagnostics, Inc, Murrieta, CA.)

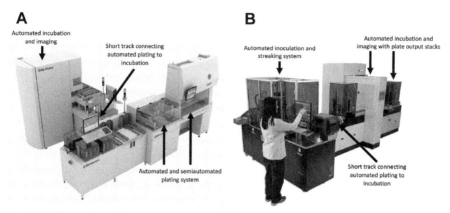

Fig. 2. (*A*) Illustration of Kiestra WCA partial laboratory automation system. (*B*) Illustration of WASPLab partial laboratory automation system. (*Courtesy of* [*A*] Becton Dickinson, Sparks, MD; and [*B*] Copan Diagnostics, Inc, Murrieta, CA.)

partial automation (**Fig. 2**); and front-end processing, plus automated incubation and imaging with a track system to deliver plates to multiple workbenches called total automation (**Fig. 3**). Distinctions among the three are important to understand because efficiency and impact on laboratory workforce are different.

Characteristics and components of Kiestra InoquIA and WASP DT automated plating systems have been reviewed and summarized multiple times and a summary of their features is available in **Table 1**.[1–7] Modules beyond up front processing include the Kiestra Work Cell Automation (WCA) and Kiestra TLA systems, and the Copan WASPLab system. **Table 2** contains a summary of Kiestra WCA and TLA, and Copan WASPLab system functions beyond automated plating. Although both systems are

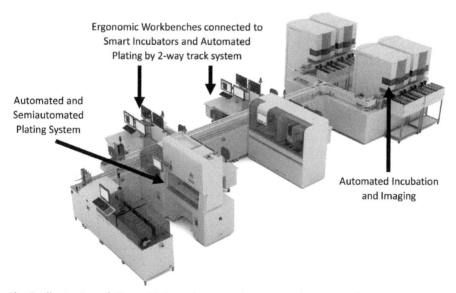

Fig. 3. Illustration of Kiestra TLA total automation system. (*Courtesy of* Becton Dickinson, Sparks, MD.)

Table 1
Comparison of Kiestra InoculA and WASP-DT automated plating systems

Feature	Kiestra InoculA	WASP-DT
Specimen types	Liquid-based, automated Nonliquid, semiautomated (manual inoculation automated streaking) Nonliquid, first inoculation (manual inoculation and streaking added to system after inoculation and streaking)	Liquid-based including sputum and stool, automated Nonliquid, streak-only mode (manual inoculation automated streaking)
Maximum capacity of specimen containers: load capacity	270 specimens loaded in 6 racks	72 specimens loaded in 12 racks (instrument allows continuous loading at any time as space becomes available)
Consumable waste: disposables	Pipette tip, beads, and plate labels	Reusable loops (30,000 inoculations/loop) and plate labels
Automatic decapping/recapping	Yes, tubes from multiple vendors	Yes, recommended to use Copan specimen containers
Number of different media that are available at one time	24	9
Plate storage	1836 plates	324–378 plates
Broth storage	5 racks of 45	4 racks of 12
Biosafety cabinet-laminar flow/HEPA filter	Yes	Yes
Continuous loading/unloading of system with specimens	Yes, with system pause	Yes
Automated sample mixing	Yes	Yes
Automated sample centrifugation	No	Yes
Method (volume) of inoculation	Pipet (10–900 µL)	Loop (1 µL, 10 µL, 30 µL), spreaders
Inoculum dispense verification	Yes	Yes
Streaking method	Rolling bead	Loop
Streaking patterns	Multiple standard and custom	Multiple standard and custom
Number of plates streaked at once	Up to 5	1
Automated broth inoculation	Yes (10–900 µL)	Yes (1 µL, 10 µL, 30 µL to Copan tubes only)
Automated biplate inoculation	Yes	Yes
Plate throughput	220 plates/h standard streaking	180 plates/h standard streaking
Specimen throughput	Depends on streaking pattern and number of plates/specimen	Depends on streaking pattern and number of plates/specimen
Slide preparation: automated smear made on glass slide	Yes	Yes

Data available at BD Kiestra and Copan Web sites. Data reviewed by respective manufacturers.

Table 2
Comparison of Kiestra WCA/TLA and WASPLab total automation systems

Feature	Kiestra WCA/TLA	WaspLab
Incubators	ReadA Compact (WCA/TLA) CO_2 and aerobic	Smart Incubators CO_2 and aerobic
Capacity	1152 plates/incubator	795 single incubator, 1590 double incubator
Imaging of plates	User defined, including 0 h	User defined, including 0 h
Imaging from multiple angles and variable lighting	Yes	Variable lighting
Camera resolution	5 MP	27 MP
Imaging throughput	Up to 300 images/h/incubator	Information not available
Workflow	Input, output, and imaging lanes with 2 elevators within each incubator	Dual robot system for moving and holding plates
Incubator throughput	300 plates/h input 300 plates/h output	Information not available
Output capacity	4 separate output stackers (boxes) per incubator	Scalable work-up canister system
Integrated track	ProceedA	Yes
Track connects automated inoculation to incubators	Yes (WCA/TLA)	Yes
Track connects incubators to output stack for work-up	Yes (WCA/TLA)	Yes
Track connects incubators to integrated workstations and integrated workstations to incubator (2-way track)	Yes (TLA)	Track connects to work-up cannister system
Ergonomic workstations	Yes, ErgonomicA (TLA) integrated into track system	Yes, ergonomic workstations free-standing
Dashboard monitor organizes current and upcoming tasks	Yes	Yes
Plate-reading software	Synapsis (WCA/TLA)	PhenoMATRIX
Colony picking	No	Yes Calibri

Data available at BD Kiestra and Copan Web sites. Data reviewed by respective manufacturers.

innovative and offer automated solutions to laboratory tasks, differences with potential impact to users do exist. Next is a list of features one should examine in both systems that may represent differences relevant to laboratory setting[8]:

- Ease of processing nonliquid specimens
- Throughput of specimens and timing of specimen arrival in the laboratory for set up
- Ease and speed of sorting and delivering inoculated plates for off-line incubation, such as anaerobic culture
- Ease of recording image analysis culture data, colonies needing further work, and interface with laboratory information system

- User organized dashboard for organizing the benchwork
- Ease of plate retrieval from the instrument to minimize technologist movement
- Ease of sorting plates following the final culture result for discard, storage, or special off-line work, such as molecular typing
- Ease of batch reporting, such as negatives, from automated system
- Automated reading of negative agar plates and chromagar plates, and autoquantitation of urine plates

WHY TOTAL AUTOMATION IN CLINICAL MICROBIOLOGY?

A key driver of total automation is labor. Surveys have shown that microbiology, along with all clinical laboratory specialties, has a shortage of technical workers that will accelerate in the near future because of high retirement rates and too few new technologists entering the profession.[1,4,9] These factors cause many clinical microbiology laboratories to be chronically understaffed with no relief in coming years. Looking at an average day in the life of a microbiology technologist, greater than 30% of time is devoted to manual tasks, such as plate and broth medium inoculation.[10] Another 10% of time is spent on transferring media to and from incubators. The NorthShore University HealthSystem clinical microbiology laboratory, which serves four hospitals and more than 100 outpatient locations, purchases approximately 700,000 bacteriology agar plates each year. During traditional bacterial culture work-up, plates are moved an average of five times between storage, incubators, benchtop, and waste. These simple but necessary moves total 3,500,000 manual plate transfers per year. Automating these processes was unthinkable until 2014 when the first fully automated bacteriology systems were installed in North America, but by reducing these time-consuming transfers we are able to save technologist time, reducing the need for laboratory workers, and effectively addressing labor shortages. This represents just one of the many documented efficiencies that have been gained with automated microbiology discussed in publications listed next:

- Reduced costs[4,11–13]
- Automating manual tasks thereby freeing technologists for more skilled responsibilities, such as microscopy, plate interpretation, and antimicrobial susceptibility testing[2,3,14]
- Improved efficiency as measured by LEAN and similar benchmarks[11,13,15]
- Reduced TATs from specimen collection to preliminary and final reports[10,16,17]
- Improved quality based on fewer processing and reporting errors[10]
- Consolidation of laboratory space[5]

THE MICROBIOLOGY LABORATORY STAFF, WILL THEY ACCEPT AUTOMATION?

The first question during the first vendor presentation in our search for an automated system was, "There are fewer workbench seats in your design for our laboratory than there are people in this room. Are we losing our jobs?" In the end, we found we needed to reduce staffing by six full-time equivalents (FTEs). Because of training, system validation, automation learning curve, and that we were the first laboratory to install the Kiestra TLA System in the United States, we negotiated with administration to attrition through the end of the second year following go-live. As a result of retirements, moving from the area, and transferring to other laboratory areas within clinical pathology, our six FTE reduction was complete, without resorting to layoffs, well before the 2-year deadline (see **Table 6**).

Did technologists accept automation?[18] Some did and some did not. One may be surprised to learn that 10 laboratories installing laboratory automation can use the system in 10 (or more) different ways. Importantly, not all 10 ways are equally efficient. The temptations to automate conventional processes, such as reading by specimen type (eg, urines, respiratory, wounds) or having the same technologist read, interpret, and work up a culture, are persuasive based on embedded manual systems and historical knowledge. Unfortunately, these processes are inefficient when combined with the tools of automation.

A key in our transformation from a conventional to an automated laboratory was the formation of a "key user group." This group met weekly, assessing problems and successes, and was instrumental in keeping the laboratory on track to achieve our goals of efficiency, accuracy, and reduced TAT. The key user group developed new processes, which were then presented weekly to the entire staff for discussion. Changes could and were made. Once finalized, everyone had to adhere to the new or changed procedures. Not surprisingly, consensus was difficult. Everyone believed their method was best. Some were reluctant to change and did not want others working on "their" cultures. Leadership, at this point, was important, emphasizing the potential gains to the laboratory and patient care. After trying a new process for 1 week, the key user group reviewed results; decided to scrap, modify, or keep as is; and then moved to the next potential process improvement. Repeating this procedure for years (it still functions 4 years after go-live, although with a less rigorous meeting schedule) created a bacteriology process that approaches plate reading and culture work-up in ways unimaginable with conventional workflow and with close to a 50% increase in the amount of work performed per technologist. Our group would never agree to return to conventional methods.

WHAT IS GAINED?
Quality: Automated Barcoding

Laboratory automation improves many quality metrics in the microbiology laboratory. Because the instrument is reading specimen barcodes, requesting assigned media based on the specimen type, labeling media with patient identifiers, and tracking plate locations throughout the automated process, laboratory-based preanalytic errors, such as mislabeling plates with the wrong patient information, selecting incorrect media, and misplacing a plate or plates, are eliminated.[5,19]

Quality: Automated Plate Inoculation and Streaking

Plate streaking is another area where laboratory automation improves quality.[5,19,20] Most cultures are plated using four quadrant or quantitative streaking methods. Results are then reported using semiquantitative modifiers (rare, few, moderate, many, or 1+, 2+, 3+, 4+) or quantitative ranges (<10,000, 10–50,000, 50–100,000, >100,000 cfu/mL). Anyone who has spent time in a traditional microbiology laboratory knows that despite attempts to standardize reporting, the output is variable among technologists. There is variation in the amount of specimen plated because of technical issues. For quantitative urine and bronchoalveolar lavage cultures, a 10-μL or 1-μL loop collects an estimated volume that can vary because of viscosity of the specimen or additional fluid adhering to the shaft that runs down adding to the inoculum. Plate streaking technique is another procedure where variability is introduced. The number of bacteria spread from one quadrant to another depends on the method used by each technologist. Large workloads with concomitant increases in stress speed the inoculating technologist through steaking patterns, resulting in poor spatial separation of colony types and limited ability to determine relative quantities of organism present.

Laboratory automation eliminates variables present with manual operation by placing a precise amount of specimen on each plate and performing the task of plate streaking exactly the same every time. Consistent automated streaking results in a clear differentiation of relative numbers of colony types with quadrant streaking and consistent estimates of colony counts with quantitative urine streaking (**Fig. 4**). This allows easier and more accurate differentiation by the technologist of potential pathogen from contaminating microbiota. Additional benefits are the decreased need for subculture to obtain pure growth for identification and antimicrobial susceptibility testing (**Table 3**).[7] Decreased TAT and fewer resources used are obvious benefits. These observations are borne out in multiple publications. A 2016 study evaluating plate streaking using the Copan Wasp compared with manual techniques found that use of automated streaking lead to a 32.2% increase in positive specimens with isolated colonies and a 3.4% increased detection of potential pathogens.[20] Two other studies comparing the WASP reusable metal loop with Kiestra rolling bead method of streaking for urine cultures found that Kiestra produced more accurate colony counts overall and was better at dispersing organisms resulting in more isolated colonies and less need to perform subculture in specimens with high colony counts.[7,21,22] In both cases, automated methods produced dramatically more discrete colonies than manual inoculation of media.

Efficiency: General

Efficiency is not automatic with the instillation of laboratory automation, but must be achieved by reevaluation of all laboratory processes and a culture of willingness to change, and change, and change until maximum benefits from automation are accomplished.[23] The key user group approach was our mechanism for change.

Implementation of laboratory automation allows technologists to spend less time on repetitive tasks with devotion of more time to skilled tasks, such as direct specimen Gram stain reading, plate reading and interpretation, and antimicrobial susceptibility testing results review.[4,13] Not only does the use of automation prevent boredom, it

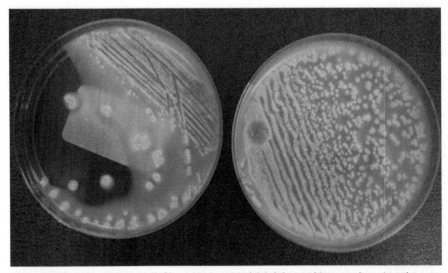

Fig. 4. Illustration of manual (*left*) and automated (*right*) streaking results using the same stool specimen and Hektoen enteric agar. Note colony separation with automated streaking.

Table 3
Comparison of manual and automated agar plate streaking (Kiestra InoculA and Copan WASP) using 41 positive urine samples processed in duplicate

Streaking Method	Subculture Needed, n (%)	Subculture Not Needed, n (%)
Manual-1	15 (37)	26 (63)
Manual-2	24 (58)	17 (42)
WASP-1	16 (39)	25 (61)
WASP-2	18 (44)	23 (56)
Inocula-1	4 (10)	37 (90)
Inocula-2	10 (24)	31 (76)

Data show that automated streaking is superior to manual streaking.[7]

also eliminates tasks resulting in repetitive movements that cause injury (**Fig. 5**). Both Kiestra TLA and WASPLab include ergonomic workbenches that provide additional protection against injury.[24,25]

Efficiency: Decreased Incubation Time Required for the Detection of Organism Growth

Incubators attached by track systems to automated inoculation instrumentation, referred to generically as "smart" incubators, decrease incubation time needed to visualize bacterial growth. Rapid growth results from immediate incubation after inoculation and eliminates plates waiting in half-filled canisters in the setup area before a stack is manually carried and loaded into a conventional incubator. Smart incubators maintain consistent temperature and gas levels as plates move in and out through a small, slim slit with negligible heat and CO_2 gas loss.[11] In addition, plates do not have to sit on the bench while work-up of other specimens takes place. Decreased incubation times allow the first plate images for culture interpretation to occur in as little as 10 hours for urine specimens and 6 hours for positive blood culture broth subcultures (**Fig. 6**).[3,26,27] The use of younger colonies for matrix-assisted laser desorption ionization time of flight (MALDI-TOF) identification and antimicrobial testing have been validated.[28] Shortened overall TAT for identification and susceptibility testing has also been documented (**Table 4**).[17]

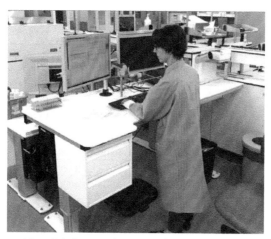

Fig. 5. Ergonomic workbench being used as a stand-up workspace.

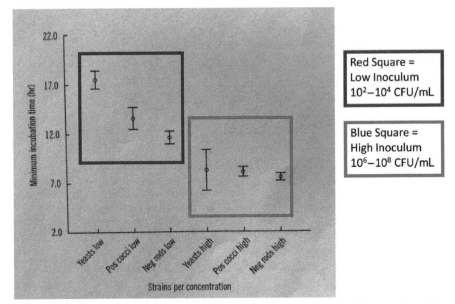

Fig. 6. Minimum incubation times needed with smart incubators to achieve colony plate growth using seeded microbial suspensions.[11] Bars indicate 95% confidence intervals.

Efficiency: 24/7 Automated Plate Inoculations and Incubation

Automated plating makes 24/7 specimen processing with plate inoculations and incubation broadly available. Studies by Burckhardt and colleagues[29] found that using laboratory automation for methicillin-resistant *Staphylococcus aureus* (MRSA) screening from nasal swabs reduced the mean reporting time from 48 hours to 20 hours, primarily by allowing them to process specimens 7 days per week rather than weekdays only. The same authors used digital plate reading to monitor the minimum amount of time needed to visualize growth on MRSA, gram-negative multidrug resisant organism (MDRO), and vancomycin-resistant enterococci. Chromogenic media and found that 20 hours was sufficient for MRSA and gram-negative MDRO detection, but because of the slow rate of bacterial growth, vancomycin-resistant enterococci screening agar needed additional imaging at 36 hours.[27]

Table 4
Reduced TATs for identification and antimicrobial susceptibility results using total laboratory automation compared with conventional processing

	Median TAT (h)		
Time to Reporting	Conventional Processing and Culture Work-Up (1330 Positive Urine Specimens)	Total Automation Processing and Culture Work-Up (1326 Positive Urine Specimens)	P value[a]
Identification	18.0 (14.7–30.7)	16.8 (14.8–23.6)	$P<.01$
Antimicrobial susceptibility result	42.3 (39.3–55.4)	40.3 (38.1–47.1)	$P<.05$

MALDI-TOF was used for identifications during both time periods.[17]
[a] P value refers to comparison of median TAT. Interquartile ranges are listed in parentheses next to respective median values.

Efficiency: Labor Savings

Labor savings with automation is perceived by many to result primarily from automation of the specimen receiving, slide preparation, and plate inoculation tasks.[2–5] Our initial vendor presentation claimed a five FTE savings in the upfront specimen processing area and a one FTE savings in the image analysis-workbench tasks area. Following go-live and process refinement by the key user group, we were surprised to find that a greater labor savings occurred in the plate reading and specimen work-up phases than in up-front processing. For culture work-up we use a two-group approach of "readers" and "workers" for lack of better descriptors. Readers interpret plate images and workers handle all manual aspects of testing. Automation allows fewer staff to read more specimens in less time by viewing images. Workers avoid time spent on manual tasks, such as moving plates in and out of the incubator, finding specific plates in a stack, marking plates for colony work-up and triaging stacks of plates for rapid or overnight phenotypic tests, and setting up antimicrobial susceptibility testing. Workers perform tasks that lead to identifications and antimicrobial susceptibility results. Plates can be segregated by task with delivery to a nearby output stacker or directly to a workbench attached to a two-way track. By focusing on efficiencies afforded by automation, the key user group reduced workbench tasks to a minimum. Emerging from this approach is the sobering realization that many traditional skills, such as colony recognition and use of biochemical profiles to identify pathogens, are no longer as essential.[30] The amount of labor required and the skills of the labor force have changed.

Efficiency: Work Flow

Efficiency is gained by restructuring conventional plate reading and work-up practices as introduced previously.[13] Although there are many ways to structure workflow with automation, simply automating the conventional process where technologists read by specimen type, and perform identification and antimicrobial susceptibility tasks on the specimens they read, misses the efficiency gains that partial and total automation can provide. Using automation, readers view agar plate images, which are deemed "ready to read" after precise incubation times designated for each specimen type by the laboratory.[31] This allows the colonies to have a predictable appearance, avoids reading plates before their required incubation is completed, and allows plates to stay in optimal incubation conditions during plate interpretations, until the moment a work-up task on an isolate begins. Because plate reading is performed on a computer monitor, it can take place anywhere inside or outside of the laboratory, which allows flexibility in laboratory design.[5] For readers, efficiency is gained because all plated media are simultaneously available for viewing. No longer is media opened and viewed one plate at a time. Automation allows simultaneous examinations of all culture plates from a specimen at one time. Additionally, several light settings are used during image capture, so with a click of the mouse hemolysis can be detected. Specimen-specific interpretations are determined by "readers" who also select colony types requiring work-up and which work-up tasks are required. Pending tasks for the "worker" are then displayed on a dashboard. The quality of automated streaking most often results in isolated colonies, in our experience, resulting in the need for only a handful of subcultures each day for all incoming specimens.[7] When a subculture plate is requested, total laboratory automation selects the agar plate, applies a label with barcode and identifiers, and delivers it to the bench for inoculation by the "worker" technologist via a track system. As tasks are completed, plates are placed on the track for reincubation for total automation or placed in an input stacker for partial automation. The simplicity and efficiency of this approach are obvious and substantiated with laboratory metrics (**Fig. 7**).

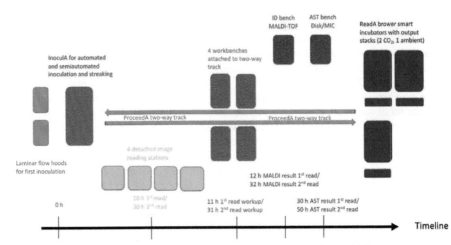

Fig. 7. Laboratory design, workflow, and turnaround times with total laboratory automation using urine as an example. AST, antimicrobial susceptibility testing; ID, identification; MALDI-TOF, matrix-assisted laser desorption/ionization -time of flight; MIC, minimum inhibitory concentration. (*Data from* NorthShore Microbiology.)

Use of the reader-worker model leads to a collaborative interpretation and work-up of cultures. Accuracy and completion of preliminary and final results belong to the group of technologists rather than to an individual. The equitable distribution of work results in no one being done until everyone is done with all specimen reading and work-up. This is in contrast to most conventional reading systems where a technologist is assigned a specimen type, such as urine, and is finished when all urine interpretations and work-up are complete. The automation model also allows a great amount of flexibility because technologists can move between being readers and workers depending on the actual workloads displayed on the dashboard. With this model two different "sets of eyes" are on every culture being worked up, resulting in strict adherence to laboratory protocols, which, in turn, improves the quality and consistency of results. Efficiency is gained by technologists being able to focus on a single task. No longer are they distracted by stacks of agar plates on their benches or running back and forth to the incubator. Dangerous and frequent plate dropping is virtually eliminated using automation.[13] Overall specimen volumes, laboratory courier arrival times, specimen incubation times, and "ready to read" times are tracked by automation software and adjusted to provide culture results at optimum technologist staffing times and, importantly, provide results when clinicians are most likely to act on results.[5] The dashboard not only tracks images ready for reading and work-up tasks pending, it also shows the number of images that will be ready for reading throughout the remainder of the day. This allows workers to plan breaks based on current and future workloads.

Measuring Efficiency

Measuring gains in efficiency is made difficult by the many variables and lack of standard measures among laboratories.[32] We found the following efficiencies when we compared the year before we went live to the 2 years following implementation of total automation:

- Overall microbiology laboratory FTEs were reduced by 22%, with a 40% reduction for bacteriology staff.

- We were able to accommodate a 17% increase in testing in the 2 years following total automation implementation with our reduced staff.
- The number of tests performed per FTE increased by 41%. This is calculated using all staff as the denominator, not just bacteriology staff.
- Supply costs attributed to culture, organism identification, and antimicrobial testing were reduced despite higher specimen volumes and annual cost increases.

Gains in efficiency will continue to improve as automated MALDI-TOF spotting and antimicrobial testing modules are incorporated into automated instrumentation.

To summarize efficiency gains, the addition of total automation combined with novel approaches to laboratory processes, including splitting the image reading and culture work-up tasks between different technologists, training all technologists to read all specimen types, and considering all cultures as one "bench" rather than separating by urine, respiratory, wounds, and so forth, has improved quality, TATs, and patient care.

Accessibility of Culture Images

Laboratory automation allows plate image capture to be scheduled at any timepoint or multiple timepoints during incubation.[2,5] Images can then be viewed on computer screens from any computer containing image analysis software. In our laboratory, this software is available on all bacteriology bench computers, the laboratory director's clinical consultation bench, and the desktop computers in the manager's and directors' office (**Fig. 8**). For some systems plate images can also be captured at will to check for growth outside of programmed times, which is convenient when answering physician queries or for curious and impatient laboratory directors that are closely following a particular culture. Images of all reading timepoints are saved and can be viewed retrospectively, which is helpful when

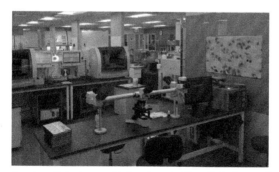

Fig. 8. Laboratory director clinical consultation bench. The clinical consultation bench is the site for intralaboratory and extralaboratory consultations. Intralaboratory consultations originate from technologists interpreting or working up specimens. They note their question in the LIS in the specimen work card and print a specimen label that is pasted to a "consultation" clipboard that is collected by the director and carried to the consultation bench. The consultation bench includes all direct specimen Gram stains filed by accession number, a computer with access to the LIS, Kiestra images, and inpatient and outpatient electronic medical records, and a multiheaded microscope with a wall mounted monitor for group viewing. Review of patient and specimen information results in an answer that is typed into the LIS specimen work card for technologist follow-up. Extralaboratory consultations from clinicians are reviewed in a similar fashion with answers typed into the patient's electronic medical record.

investigating physician questions after plates have become overgrown or discarded.

Safety

Laboratory automation dramatically reduces the number of agar plates being handled by technologists on a daily basis. A total of 3.5 million manual plate movements were eliminated in our laboratory each year, and many of these agar plates contain bacterial colonies. Automation moves plates to the technologist or to an output stacker, but not every culture plate, only the one plate on which isolate work-up is being performed (eg, only the MacConkey agar for identification of a gram-negative rod). This results in less spread of bacteria around the microbiology laboratory because of accidental (noticed and unnoticed) touching of organism and dropped plates. Because all plates from a culture are viewed at the same time on one screen, there is less opportunity for surprises, such as opening a plate on the workbench with a mold colony or possible bioterrorism organisms. Although proper biosafety procedures should always be followed, laboratory automation minimizes surprises that represent exposure risk.[13]

WHAT IS LOST?
Technical Knowledge and Skills

The successful introduction of automation in the microbiology laboratory is not without loss of technical knowledge and manual skills that were acquired through decades of experience with conventional methods.[2,30] In addition to needing fewer staff, skills needed by technologists with automation are different. Experience with plate steaking, reliance on biochemical and physical tests for identification, colony recognition, and plate bacterial Gram stain morphologies are less necessary with automation. However, visual pattern recognition of the relative numbers of pathogen verses specimen commensals present on agar surfaces, understanding of new and expanding taxonomic names that are associated with specific diseases, antimicrobial susceptibility testing methods and their interpretation, and comfort and competence with computer software and instrumentation are emphasized in an automated laboratory.

Pride and Ownership Associated with Conventional Workflow

Traditional workflow approaches and the use of conventional methods have been the mainstay of clinical microbiology successes for decades. A technologist reads and interprets a culture plate and follows with necessary identification and antimicrobial tests to finish test results for the day. The "stamp of approval" for this set of results is one person's responsibility. Dividing this responsibility between two or more technologists can introduce a loss of ownership. Technologists trained in the conventional tradition may find it difficult to transition to an automated, multitechnologist per specimen work-up system. In support of automation, multiple technologists viewing one culture and agreeing on one interpretation are a strong support for clear laboratory procedures, technologist training, and consistent technologist performance. This is the essence of quality improvement.

Day Shift–Only Plate Reading

The automated microbiology laboratory has different technologist work schedules. As laboratories have become a 7-day-per-week workplace to accommodate contemporary hospital reimbursement models, so they will become a 24/7 workplace with automation because of improved quality, and pay for performance and capitation reimbursement models.[33] The availability of images for interpretation throughout evening and overnight shifts and the early set-up of identification and antimicrobial tests can dramatically reduce TATs for hospitalized patients' results. The ability to confirm an infectious diagnosis and etiology, finalize therapeutic decisions, or rule out infection with a negative culture reduces additional testing and speeds up discharge management. Creativity with the timing of results reporting is in the early stages of experimentation. Plate reading 24/7 with total automation will redefine results reporting and once shorter TATs are known to be available there will be no stopping progress toward all that automation can offer (**Fig. 9**).[30,34]

Automation Downtime

Without automation there is no worry about unanticipated system failure and downtime. Once automated, it is immediately recognized that downtime with automation is different than downtime with an automated blood culture system or identification/ Antimicrobiol Susceptibility Test system. If automation fails, inoculations, incubations, culture interpretation, and work-up stop. Rather than one blood culture technologist stymied in their activity, the whole laboratory does not function. Fortunately, full system failure is extremely rare, and when it does happen, field service representatives are responsive by telephone or are physically present.[4,5] Luckily, with total or partial automation, failure of a component does not result in failure of full automation. If the inoculation system is down, incubation, imaging, and plate retrieval still function. There are workarounds one can use, such as manual inoculation and uploading plates into the incubator. The usual automation interruptions are minor or planned preventive maintenance procedures (**Table 5**). Both of these can be scheduled in advance at a time that is most convenient for the laboratory, most often the slowest time of the day, and generally last from minutes to a few hours (**Boxes 1** and **2**).

What skills need to be retained for automation down time? Conventional skills are diminished or lost with laboratory automation. Down time occurrences do not require a full return to conventional procedures. When a component or components of an automated system are unavailable because of a planned or unanticipated down time, such skills as manual plate steaking are needed. This allows incubation, growth, identification, and antimicrobial testing to be performed off-line in emergency situations. In the end, what the traditional microbiology technologist might miss the most is the smell of volatile microbial metabolites that gives every conventional laboratory its familiar smell. The

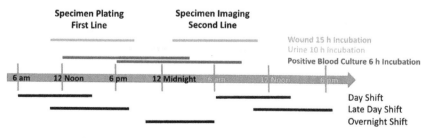

Fig. 9. Adjusting technologist readers and bench workers to automation workflow based on specimen volumes, courier schedules, specimen incubation, and ready-to-read times. Note overlapping technologist scheduling that allows interpreting images and culture work-up 24/7. (*Data from* NorthShore Microbiology).

Table 5
Most common Kiestra TLA error alarms and time to resolve (NorthShore data)

Error Information	Location within Kiestra TLA of Error Alarm			
	BarcodA (Plate Labeling)	InoqulA (Inoculation and Streaking)	ProceedA (Track)	ReadA Compacts (Smart Incubators)
Error (cause of error)	Label not sticking (moist plate)	Pipette tip held too long (failure to read label)	Time out (dirty sensor)	Suction cup did not lift lid (cracked lid)
Time to resolve, min	<2	<5	<2	<2

automated laboratory is odor-free, quiet, and relaxed. Perhaps not so difficult to get used to?

WHO CAN AFFORD AUTOMATION?
Return on Investment

Laboratory automation for microbiology is not free. There is an initial capital cost for instrumentation and ongoing service contracts. Laboratory renovation is another cost. So, who can afford laboratory automation and how can you make the case for affordability at your institution?

Hard or direct cost savings is dominated by the use of fewer laboratory FTEs to accomplish the same amount of work with automation. Calculations for return on investment based on our (NorthShore) labor savings are shown in **Table 6**.

Total Automation Occupies Less Space

Expanding the use of molecular platforms in microbiology underscores the need for more laboratory space. Automation allows more bacteriology processing and plate reading procedures to occur in a smaller space. We found that the multibench conventional bacteriology system required approximately 25% more space than the Kiestra totally automated system that processes 17% more work. This is accomplished by more efficient use of incubator and workbench spaces and by the need for fewer workers.

Can You Afford Not to Automate?

As laboratory reimbursement continues to transition from fee-for-service to pay for performance and capitation models, emphasis will fall on laboratories to reduce cost, improve efficiency and quality, and impact patient care by providing more rapid results.[33] In our setting, based on the TAT reduction for positive and negative culture results, and AST result, total automation was credited by our corporate finance department with an additional $245,000 annual savings based on earlier discharge and improved hospital bed management. Taken together, cost savings reflected in labor ($468,750) and reduced reported TATs ($245,000) provided approximately

Box 1
Troubleshooting unplanned downtime, periodic controls NorthShore data

Technologist trained: fixes 90% of problems

On-line BD iPad or telephone support: fixes 6% of problems

BD field service engineer: fixes 4% of problems

Box 2
Periodic controls and scheduled preventive maintenance for Kiestra TLA (NorthShore data)

Daily: known concentration of bacterial suspensions × 2 and sterile broth × 1

Weekly: general topical cleaning

Quarterly: ReadA compact (smart incubators) cleaning and calibration

Periodic: BD scheduled preventive maintenance

$700,000 annual savings and a return on investment of 3 rather than 5 (labor savings only) years (see **Table 6**). Additional savings are achieved through expense management shown by flat microbiology laboratory costs despite 3.5% annual CPI increases; increased productivity, which in our laboratory resulted in a 41% increase in tests/FTE; and positive impacts of quality and speed on antimicrobial stewardship. Although MALDI-TOF cost justification may have been the easiest and most convincing ever for microbiology leadership, total automation is close behind. With a financially more competitive future in view, how can one afford not automate?

THE FUTURE AND ADDITIONAL GAINS OF AUTOMATION IN MICROBIOLOGY

The automated microbiology laboratory will continue to improve quality, efficiency, and TATs.[1] Improvements that are expected to appear in the near future include automated reading of no-growth plates, automated plate quantitative counts, automated colony recognition and differentiation with chromagar plates, automated MALDI-TOF target spotting, and antimicrobial susceptibility testing including disk diffusion reading and reporting.[2,14] The eventual mating of automated blood culture instrumentation with total automation is also being planned. Complete automation of bacteriology procedures using systems that are modular introduces the distinct possibility that laboratory consolidation will take on a new and improved paradigm, remote, automated bacterial processing with central core laboratory image interpretation.[35,36] Although the impact of automation is compelling, we have merely scratched the surface of what the future of automated clinical microbiology could be.

Table 6
Labor savings with total automation that impacted return on investment (NorthShore data)

Date	FTEs Lost (Attrition)	FTE Gained
September, 2013	1.0	
January, 2014	0.2	
June, 2014	1.0	
October, 2014	1.0	
December, 2014 (TLA Go-Live)	1.8	0.3
March, 2015	1.0	
April, 2015		0.8
July, 2015		1.0
August, 2015	2.1	
Totals	8.1 lost	2.1 gained
Net	6.0 FTEs lost	

2014 data: average wage $62,500 + average fringe $15,625 = $78,125. $78,125 (total cost/FTE) × 6 FTEs lost = $468,750 annual savings.

REFERENCES

1. Bourbeau PP, Ledeboer NA. Automation in clinical microbiology. J Clin Microbiol 2013;51(6):1658–65.
2. Bailey A, Ledeboer N, Burnham C-AD. Clinical microbiology is growing up: the total laboratory automation revolution. Clin Chem 2018. https://doi.org/10.1373/clinchem.2017.274522.
3. Burckhardt I. Laboratory automation in clinical microbiology. Bioengineering (Basel) 2018;5(4) [pii:E102].
4. Novak SM, Marlowe EM. Automation in the clinical microbiology laboratory. Clin Lab Med 2013;33(3):567–88.
5. Croxatto A, Prod'hom G, Faverjon F, et al. Laboratory automation in clinical bacteriology: what system to choose? Clin Microbiol Infect 2016;22(3):217–35.
6. Greub G, Prod'hom G. Automation in clinical bacteriology: what system to choose? Clin Microbiol Infect 2011;17(5):655–60.
7. Croxatto A, Dijkstra K, Prod'hom G, et al. Comparison of inoculation with the InoqulA and WASP automated systems with manual inoculation. J Clin Microbiol 2015;53(7):2298–307.
8. Burnham C-AD, Dunne WM, Greub G, et al. Automation in the clinical microbiology laboratory. Clin Chem 2013;59(12):1696–702.
9. Garcia E, Kundu I, Ali A, et al. The American Society for Clinical Pathology's 2016-2017 vacancy survey of medical laboratories in the United States. Am J Clin Pathol 2018;149:387–400.
10. Dauwalder O, Landrieve L, Laurent F, et al. Does bacteriology laboratory automation reduce time to results and increase quality management? Clin Microbiol Infect 2016;22(3):236–43.
11. Mutters NT, Hodiamont CJ, De Jong MD, et al. Performance of Kiestra total laboratory automation combined with MS in clinical microbiology practice. Ann Lab Med 2014;34(2):111–7.
12. Archetti C, Montanelli A, Finazzi D, et al. Clinical laboratory automation: a case study. J Public Health Res 2017;6(1). https://doi.org/10.4081/jphr.2017.881.
13. Da Rin G, Zoppelletto M, Lippi G. Integration of diagnostic microbiology in a model of total laboratory automation. Lab Med 2016;47(1):73–82.
14. Croxatto A, Marcelpoil R, Orny C, et al. Towards automated detection, semi-quantification and identification of microbial growth in clinical bacteriology: a proof of concept. Biomed J 2017;40(6):317–28.
15. Samuel L, Novak-Weekley S. The role of the clinical laboratory in the future of health care: lean microbiology. J Clin Microbiol 2014;52(6):1812–7.
16. Graham M, Tilson L, Streitberg R, et al. Improved standardization and potential for shortened time to results with BD Kiestra total laboratory automation of early urine cultures: a prospective comparison with manual processing. Diagn Microbiol Infect Dis 2016;86(1):1–4.
17. Theparee T, Das S, Thomson RB. Total laboratory automation and matrix-assisted laser desorption ionization-time of flight mass spectrometry improve turnaround times in the clinical microbiology laboratory: a retrospective analysis. J Clin Microbiol 2018;56(1) [pii:e01242-17].
18. McAlearney AS, Hefner JL, Sieck CJ, et al. The journey through grief: insights from a qualitative study of electronic health record implementation. Health Serv Res 2015;50(2):462–88.
19. Murray PR. Laboratory automation: efficiency and turnaround times. Microbiol Aust 2014;35(1):49.

20. Quiblier C, Jetter M, Rominski M, et al. Performance of Copan WASP for routine urine microbiology. Onderdonk AB, ed. J Clin Microbiol 2016;54(3):585–92.
21. Iversen J, Stendal G, Gerdes CM, et al. Comparative evaluation of inoculation of urine samples with the Copan WASP and BD Kiestra InoqulA instruments. Lede-boer NA, ed. J Clin Microbiol 2016;54(2):328–32.
22. Froment P, Marchandin H, Vande Perre P, et al. Automated versus manual sample inoculations in routine clinical microbiology: a performance evaluation of the fully automated InoqulA instrument. J Clin Microbiol 2014;52(3):796–802.
23. Yarbrough ML, Lainhart W, McMullen AR, et al. Impact of total laboratory automa-tion on workflow and specimen processing time for culture of urine specimens. Eur J Clin Microbiol Infect Dis 2018;37(12):2405–11.
24. Shrestha N, Kukkonen-Harjula KT, Verbeek JH, et al. Workplace interventions for reducing sitting at work. Cochrane Database Syst Rev 2018;(6):CD010912. https://doi.org/10.1002/14651858.CD010912.pub4.
25. Hoe VC, Urquhart DM, Kelsall HL, et al. Ergonomic design and training for preventing work-related musculoskeletal disorders of the upper limb and neck in adults. Cochrane Database Syst Rev 2012;(8):CD008570. https://doi.org/10.1002/14651858.CD008570.pub2.
26. De Socio GV, Di Donato F, Paggi R, et al. Laboratory automation reduces time to report of positive blood cultures and improves management of patients with bloodstream infection. Eur J Clin Microbiol Infect Dis 2018;37(12):2313–22.
27. Burckhardt I, Last K, Zimmermann S. Shorter incubation times for detecting multi-drug resistant bacteria in patient samples: defining early imaging time points us-ing growth kinetics and total laboratory automation. Ann Lab Med 2019;39:43–9.
28. Curtoni A, Cipriani R, Marra ES, et al. Rapid identification of microorganisms from positive blood culture by MALDI-TOF MS after short-term incubation on solid me-dium. Curr Microbiol 2017;74(1):97–102.
29. Burckhardt I, Horner S, Burckhardt F, et al. Detection of MRSA in nasal swabs: marked reduction of time to report for negative reports by substituting classical manual workflow with total lab automation. Eur J Clin Microbiol Infect Dis 2018;37(9):1745–51.
30. Ledeboer NA, Dallas SD. The automated clinical microbiology laboratory: fact or fantasy? J Clin Microbiol 2014;52(9):3140–6.
31. Rhoads DD, Novak SM, Pantanowitz L. A review of the current state of digital plate reading of cultures in clinical microbiology. J Pathol Inform 2015;6:23.
32. Lewis MR, Bryant RJ. Benchmarking and performance monitoring: what is appropriate for your laboratory?. In: Garcia LS, editor. Clinical laboratory man-agement. 2nd edition. Washington, DC: American Society of Microbiology; 2014. p. 890–4. https://doi.org/10.1128/9781555817282.ch50.
33. O'Brien JM, Kumar A, Metersky ML. Does value-based purchasing enhance quality of care and patient outcomes in the ICU? Crit Care Clin 2013;29(1):91–112.
34. Greatorex J, Ellington MJ, Koser CU, et al. New methods for identifying infectious diseases. Br Med Bull 2014;112(1):27–35.
35. Matthews S, Deutekom J. The future of diagnostic bacteriology. Clin Microbiol Infect 2011;17(5):651–4.
36. Mascart G, Martiny D, Miendje Y, et al. Automatisation en bactériologie: quel ave-nir ? Un exemple concret dans le cadre d'une consolidation de laboratoires uni-versitaires. Ann Biol Clin (Paris) 2018;76(4):365–72.

Matrix-Assisted Laser Desorption/Ionization Time-of-Flight: The Revolution in Progress

Alexandra L. Bryson, PhD[a], Emily M. Hill, PhD[b],
Christopher D. Doern, PhD[a],*

KEYWORDS

- MALDI-TOF MS • Infectious diseases diagnostics • Rapid organism identification
- Phenotypic susceptibility testing

KEY POINTS

- Extraction methods for mycobacteria and fungi require standardization and are critical to optimizing matrix-assisted laser desorption/ionization time-of-flight mass spectrometry (MALDI-TOF MS) performance.
- Rapid, phenotypic, growth-based susceptibility testing methods for MALDI-TOF MS have been developed for both gram-positive and gram-negative bacteria, as well as yeast.
- Several novel methods for rapid organism identification from positive blood cultures have been developed and include direct-from-bottle identification as well as short-incubation identification.
- Significant progress has been made in the use of MALDI-TOF MS for the direct identification of organisms from preculture urine specimens.

INTRODUCTION

Matrix-assisted laser desorption/ionization time-of-flight mass spectrometry (MALDI-TOF MS) has undoubtedly changed the way clinical microbiology laboratories (CMLs) diagnose infectious diseases. Now commonly used for the routine identification of cultured bacteria and yeast, CMLs are looking to expand the use of MALDI-TOF MS to other areas of infectious diseases diagnostics. The relative ease of performance, low cost per test, and rapidity of results has prompted the development of advanced techniques, such as antimicrobial susceptibility, direct-from-specimen organism identification, and several other techniques that may improve on conventional techniques.

Disclosure: The authors have nothing to disclose.
[a] Department of Pathology, Virginia Commonwealth University Health System, 403 North 13th Street, Richmond, VA 23298, USA; [b] Pathology & Laboratory Medicine, Hunter Holmes McGuire VA Medical Center, 1201 Broad Rock Boulevard, Richmond, VA 23224, USA
* Corresponding author.
E-mail address: Christopher.doern@vcuhealth.org

Clin Lab Med 39 (2019) 391–404
https://doi.org/10.1016/j.cll.2019.05.010
0272-2712/19/© 2019 Elsevier Inc. All rights reserved.

labmed.theclinics.com

This review discusses the progress that has been made in developing MALDI-TOF MS applications beyond conventional identification of bacteria and yeast.

ADVANCES IN ORGANISM IDENTIFICATION
Identification of Mycobacteria

Traditionally, mycobacterial isolates from acid-fast bacilli (AFB)–positive cultures have been identified using phenotypic techniques.[1] These methods are time-consuming, labor intensive, and often yield erroneous results prompting the need for repeat testing. Molecular methods are technically complex, expensive, and mostly used in reference laboratories.[2] In contrast, MALDI-TOF MS is now routinely used in CMLs for the identification of bacterial isolates and ongoing research is expanding the technology to identify mycobacteria; however, uniform procedures for strain inactivation and protein extraction have yet to be optimized for routine use.[3]

In contrast to bacterial identification, extraction method is critical for accurate identification of mycobacteria with MALDI-TOF MS. Therefore, over the past 10 years, several studies have sought to evaluate, standardize, and optimize the inactivation and protein extraction protocols for AFB to obtain reliable spectra for analysis.[2–4] Widespread adoption of MALDI-TOF MS for routine identification of AFB in clinical laboratories is possible with the use of manufacturer's kits for sample preparation (eg, the VITEK MS Mycobacteria/Nocardia [bioMérieux, Marcy-l'Étoile, France] and Bruker [Billerica, MA] Mycoex kits)[3,4] with analysis in duplicate or triplicate recommended and often necessary for these systems.[5] Some groups have attempted to further optimize protocols by incorporating freezing-based protein extraction, or even more efficient automatic homogenizers to rupture the mycobacteria cell wall without damaging proteins.[2]

Luo and colleagues[3] evaluated the VITEK MS v3.0 database in combination with the VITEK MS Mycobacterium/Nocardia Kit for the identification of clinically relevant Mycobacterium species. Of the 507 Mycobacterium species tested (46 Mycobacterium tuberculosis complex and 461 nontuberculous Mycobacteria [NTM]), 93.9% were correctly identified. Body and colleagues[4] in a separate study found similar results. These data suggest that adoption of the standardized sample processing kit in conjunction with the knowledge base can accurately identify mycobacteria. Of note, all Mycobacterium abscessus subspecies abscessus and massiliense were identified as M abscessus, and all Mycobacterium fortuitum, Mycobacterium senegalense, Mycobacterium peregrinum, and Mycobacterium septicum were identified as M. fortuitum group. Although MALDI-TOF MS can reliably identify M tuberculosis at the complex level, it is unable to further differentiate members within the complex.[3,5,6] Importantly, this system could reliably identify isolates grown on solid media (94%) or from liquid Mycobacterium Growth Indicator Tubes (MGIT) media (91%) with greater than 99% confidence. Conversely, Saramis v4.12 RUO identified only 67% of isolates from Middlebrook 7H10% and 62% from liquid media.[7]

Although the general principals of the currently available Bruker Daltonics (Biotyper) and BioMérieux (Vitek MS) MALDI-TOF systems are similar, the depth of their mycobacteria databases is significantly different[5] and should be carefully evaluated before purchase.[5] Furthermore, sample preparation methods, instrumentation platforms, and commercial databases have proven not to be interachangeable.[8,9]

Filamentous Fungi

Historically, the identification of filamentous fungi has been a slow and labor-intensive process that relied on the observation of morphologic features for organism identification. Therefore, commercial databases for filamentous fungi have been developed to facilitate implementation of this technology for mold identification in routine clinical settings and there is an ongoing effort to improve accuracy and reliability of this technique.[8,10]

Stein and colleagues[10] evaluated 3 MALDI-TOF MS libraries for the identification of filamentous fungi in 3 laboratories using the Bruker Microflex MALDI-TOF MS instrument. Identifications obtained by the Bruker Mold Library, National Institutes of Health (NIH) Library, and Mass Spectrometry Identification (MSI) online library were compared with both conventional and molecular identification methods. Of the 221 mold isolates tested, the highest rate of species-level identification (72%) was obtained with MSI, followed by 19.5% with NIH, and 13.6% with Bruker. Due to library limitations and/or imperfect spectra, more than 20% of the molds included in the study remained unidentified to the species level with all 3 libraries. Identification rates to the genus level were 33.5% with Bruker and 50.2% with the NIH library.[10]

A multicenter evaluation of the Vitek MS v3.0 system for the identification of 26 genera including 51 species of filamentous fungi correctly identified 91% of isolates. An additional 2% of isolates identified correctly at the genus level. Seven percent were misidentified either due to incorrect identification or reporting of multiple genera. Vitek MS accurately identified 100% of dimorphic fungi, 93% of *Aspergillus* to the specie level, 86% of *Mucorales* to species level, and 85% of dermatophytes to the species level. Like other reports, dermatophytes, in particular, the *Trichophyton* species, proved difficult to accurately identify.[10,11]

With the Bruker system, acceptable score thresholds for reliable organism identification have been established; however, these thresholds may not be appropriate for the identification of filamentous fungi. Several studies have modified these scores to improve performance. Due to the variability in technique and lack of standardized sample processing protocols, one group recommends the use of 4 spots when testing isolates and only accepting the spot with the highest score. This practice, in theory, should improve the reliability of results and improve overall performance.[12]

ADVANCES IN ANTIMICROBIAL SUSCEPTIBILITY TESTING

Several approaches have been explored for antimicrobial susceptibility testing (AST). Early efforts were primarily focused on the detection of beta-lactamase activity and cell wall changes in gram-negative bacteria. Although the analytical performance of these techniques appears to be acceptable, they are labor-intensive and as a result, have not been widely adopted. The more compelling applications include detection of resistance markers such as altered penicillin binding protein PBP2a', which confers methicillin resistance in staphylococci, or the presence of carbapenemases in gram-negative bacilli. These techniques may provide critical resistance information at the time of organism identification.

Here we solely review MALDI-TOF–based AST measurements, although there are several other MS methods, such as liquid chromatographic (LC-MS) and electron spray ionization (ESI-MS), which are being investigated. Also, detection of beta-lactamase activity through measurement of antibiotic hydrolysis products are summarized in recent reviews and are not discussed.[13]

Detection of Staphylococcal Methicillin Resistance

The detection of methicillin resistance in staphylococci dramatically changes how a patient's infection will be managed. Methicillin resistance is most frequently conferred by the production of an alternative penicillin binding protein (PBP2a'), which is encoded by the *mecA* gene. Several strategies have been used to rapidly define methicillin resistance using MALDI-TOF MS. Some of the earliest methods suggested that there were spectral patterns within the 2000-DA to 20,000-Da range that could be used to differentiate methicillin-resistant *Staphylococcus aureus* (MRSA) from methicillin-susceptible *S aureus* (MSSA).

In a recent investigation, Rhoads and colleagues[14] focused on the detection of a 2415 *m/z* peak of phenol soluble modulin molecule (PSM-mec), which is encoded within the staphylococcal cassette chromosome *mec* (SCC*mec*) types II, II, and VIII. When present, this molecule correlates with methicillin resistance in staphylococci and could potentially be used to rapidly differentiate MRSA from MSSA[14]; however, the imperfect negative predictive value limits the clinical utility of the assay.

Detection of Reduced Vancomycin Susceptibility in Staphylococcus aureus

Vancomycin therapy is a mainstay treatment for MRSA infections; however, laboratory methods for accurately detecting reduced vancomycin susceptibility perform with variable accuracy. A significant challenge is detecting vancomycin-intermediate *S aureus* (VISA) and heterogeneous vancomycin-intermediate *S aureus* (hVISA) where practical and reliable laboratory methods do not exist. To solve this problem, some have explored the use of MALDI-TOF MS for the classification of VISA and hVISA strains. For example, using a machine learning algorithm coupled with a formic acid tube extraction method, Asakura and colleagues[15] were able to quickly and accurately differentiate VISA from vancomycin-susceptible strains. Surprisingly, the method also performed well for hVISA classification and correctly identified 106 of 107 hVISA strains.

Growth-Based Susceptibility Testing of Bacteria

Mechanistic detection of resistance may not accurately detect phenotypic resistance. Thus, an appealing alternative is to use MALD-TOF to detect altered growth as an indicator of antibiotic activity. Such methods have been in development by Bruker Daltonics and are referred to as the "MALDI Biotyper antibiotic susceptibility test rapid assay" or MBT-ASTRA.

In this assay the relative amounts of growth in the presence of antibiotic is compared with growth without antibiotic during an abbreviated incubation step of approximately 2 hours. In each growth experiment, the matrix is spiked with a quantified reference standard, which allows for data normalization, and area under the curve (AUC) calculation. Higher AUCs indicate more growth and therefore antibiotic resistance. The MBT-ASTRA technique has 2 primary advantages over other MALDI-TOF MS–based resistance measurements. First, it can provide meaningful information regarding the relative susceptibility of an organism. Second, it can potentially be applied to any organism that can be reliably cultured with promising results for common gram-negative and gram-positive pathogens. Some examples of interest include meropenem susceptibility in *Klebsiella pneumoniae* with a 1-hour incubation with 64 μg/mL of antibiotic.[16] Of 36 meropenem-resistant and 72 meropenem-susceptible strains, MBT-ASTRA assay categorized 5 as falsely resistant, and 1 as falsely susceptible. Although promising, the resistant strains were *K pneumoniae* carbapenemase producers, and it is unknown how well the assay would perform with other carbapenem resistance mechanisms. Some studies have also shown promise for fastidious organisms such as gram-negative anaerobes and *Pasteurella multocida*,[17,18] *Candida* spp, and mycobacteria AST (discussed later in this article).

Stable Isotope Susceptibility Testing

In a variant on MBT-ASTRA, isotopically labeled nutrients are added to growth media.[14] Growing organisms (ie, non–antibiotic inhibited) incorporate these isotopes into bacterial mass resulting in peak shifts detected by MALDI-TOF. A proof-of-principal study demonstrated accurate prediction of tobramycin, meropenem, and ciprofloxacin susceptibility for *Pseudomonas aeruginosa*,[19] whereas in a separate effort, methicillin-resistant and MSSA were differentiated within 4 hours.[20,21] As a metabolic assay, the isotopic assay theoretically may offer earlier readout than the growth-dependent MBT-ASTRA.

Direct-on-Target Microdroplet Growth Assay

Another intriguing approach relies on detection threshold as a surrogate for antibiotic effect. Incubation occurs in small volumes applied directly to the MALDI-TOF MS target plate. Matrix is then added, and growth is scored as positive if there were sufficient organisms for an identification. In initial studies, a 4-hour to 5-hour incubation in 6-µL volume was sufficient for accurate susceptibility determinations for *K pneumoniae* and *P aeruginosa*, respectively.[21] However, studies with *Acinetobacter* only yielded less than 80% agreement with conventional minimum inhibitory concentration (MIC) methods.[22] An adaptation has also been explored for rapid AST from positive blood cultures by spotting 6-µL droplets of blood culture broth diluted into growth medium at an approximate Clinical and Laboratory Standards Institute (CLSI) standard 5×10^5/mL inoculum density. One experiment tested meropenem-resistant Enterobacteriaceae spiked into aerobic Bactec blood culture bottles.[23] Extraction of positive blood culture broth by lysis/centrifugation was determined to offer a favorable 91.7% to 92.3% sensitivity and 100% specific for detection of carbapenem resistance.

Growth-Based Susceptibility Testing of Fungi

In the past decade, proof-of-concept studies have evaluated and found promising results for rapid fluconazole[24] and echinocandin susceptibility testing of *Candida*.[25] The studies used composite correlation indexes (CCIs) to assess antifungal susceptibility, based on comparison of spectra after incubation with varying concentrations of antifungal agents. The concentrations tested are strategic; a no-drug control serves as a reference; intermediate concentrations tested are the lowest needed to confer a detectable proteomic change in a susceptible strain; whereas high concentrations tested produce significant proteomic changes in susceptible strains. The CCI compares intermediate drug concentration to the no-drug and the high-drug controls. Susceptible strains demonstrate proteomic changes more like high-drug controls, whereas resistant strains resemble no-drug controls. Three-hour incubation caspofungin susceptibility results correlated with the *fks1* echinocandin resistance mutation and were as accurate as conventional 24-hour incubation antifungal susceptibility testing. Four-hour CCI-based fluconazole susceptibility testing of *Candida tropicalis* also showed excellent essential agreement with reference methods.[26] These methods will need to be further refined to enhance reproducibility before routine clinical use.[27]

CCI has proven less tractable for evaluation of filamentous fungi such as *Aspergillus fumigatus* and *Aspergillus flavus* susceptibility to caspofungin.[28] Resistance is rare; therefore, performance is harder to evaluate, although *Aspergillus* spp susceptibility to voriconazole was found to correlate with Cyp51A-based sequence analysis. However, the 48-hour incubation thus far provides little advantage over conventional broth microdilution.[29]

The very similar, MBT-ASTRA, as described for antibacterial susceptibility testing, has been applied to antifungal susceptibility testing.[30] Rapid performance (7 hours) was excellent for *Candida albicans* (100% categorical agreement with the CLSI reference method), but less promising for *Candida glabrata* whereby there were unacceptable 5.8% very major and 20% major error rates, suggesting great potential for speeding up candidal AST, but needing further refinement.

Growth-Based Susceptibility Testing of Mycobacteria

Perhaps the AST area most in need of improved turnaround time is for mycobacteria where conventional testing requires up to several weeks. MTB ASTRA[31] (isoniazid, rifampin, and ethambutol) applied to strains of *M tuberculosis* complex AST showed 100% categorical agreement with gold standard testing; albeit, without faster turnaround time. In contrast, applied to NTM strains, it provided 98.5% categorical agreement (rifabutin, clarithromycin); however, with results available a week earlier than the gold standard. These latter promising results suggest future application for direct AST on MGIT positive for NTM.

ADVANCES IN ORGANISM IDENTIFICATION FROM CLINICAL SPECIMENS
Direct Organism Identification from Positive Blood Cultures

It is critical for laboratories to rapidly identify the causative agents of sepsis so treatment can be narrowed or optimized. Most organisms will grow and signal positive in automated blood culture systems within 2 days, and definitive organism identification requires an additional 24 to 48 hours to isolate and classify colonies. MALDI-TOF offers the ability to identify a wide range of pathogens to the genus or species level directly from positive blood culture rapidly, and at low cost. However, blood and media components, like hemoglobin and resin, create spectral noise, interfering with spectral matches with MALDI-TOF MS libraries.[32–34] Two approaches have been developed to address this issue. The first is to inoculate positive blood culture broth to solid media, incubate for 2 to 6 hours, then use MALDI-TOF MS to identify the low-level growth.[35–39] The second is to purify organism from the positive blood culture broth prior to MALDI-TOF MS identification.

Short-Incubation Matrix-assisted Laser Desorption/Ionization Time-of-Flight Mass Spectrometry

Short-incubation MALDI-TOF MS is simple and cheap. The short-incubation growth is spotted on the MALDI-TOF MS target plate for identification. One study found that the mean incubation needed to establish a genus-level identification was 2.0 hours for gram-negative bacteria and 5.9 hours for gram-positive bacteria.[35] Another reported that a 5-hour subculture allowed identification of monomicrobial blood cultures.[36] Short-incubation strategies have been less successful for anaerobic bacteria, whereby a 4-hour to 6-hour incubation only allowed organism identification less than 50% of the time.[38,39] This faster method of organism identification has been shown to improve appropriate antibiotic therapy for patients.[40]

Organism Identification Directly from Positive Blood Culture Broth

Most organism purification protocols from positive blood culture broth use varying combinations of lysis of human cells, centrifugation steps to pellet microorganisms, multiple wash steps, filtration, and protein extraction. One commercially available option is the MBT Sepsityper kit (Bruker), currently IVD-CE marked in Europe. A relatively consistent finding across purification methods is that the spectra differ from organisms grown on solid media, leading to lower MALDI-TOF MS scores (Bruker MS instruments) and confidence levels (VITEK MS). For Bruker MS instruments, the package insert recommends using scores ≥ 2.0 for species-level identification and ≥ 1.7 for genus-level identification from solid media. However, the positive blood culture literature supports ≥ 1.7 for species-level and ≥ 1.4 for genus-level identification as sufficient.[37,41–43] The blood culture bottle brand has not been reported to impact identification.[44]

The Sepsityper workflow consists of approximately 30 minutes of hands-on time, and the reagents are cheaper than molecular-based blood culture diagnostics, but can be more expensive than in-house organism purification methods.[45,46] Studies have estimated cost per sample at $5 to $9.[46,47] A large meta-analysis of the Sepsityper kit literature analyzing in aggregate 3320 monomicrobial blood cultures found correct species ID for 80% of samples: 90% for gram-negatives; 76% for gram-positives and 66% for yeast.[41] Cutoff scores used were greater than 1.7, but in some studies were not indicated.

Alternatively, multiple studies describe successful use of serum separator tubes to isolate microorganisms before MALDI-TOF identification. The method involves isolating bacteria from the top of the separating gel after centrifugation and several washing steps afterward to remove lysed red cells and debris, which can require approximately 30 minutes for processing.[43,45,48,49] Impressively, this purification technique provided 99% gram-negative identification accuracy with 96% of samples having scores ≥ 2.0. The same extraction protocol did not work as well for gram-positives. An additional protein extraction step improved results with performance equivalent to the Sepsityper method. Therefore, gram-positives appear to be more challenging with custom or commercial methods. However, cutoff scores as low as 1.4 still provided accurate identification, and with this lower threshold were able to correctly identify 87% to 90% of gram-positive pathogens.[48]

The hands-on time is a substantial barrier to implementing organism purification methods. Simon and colleagues[42] recently reported a 10-minute processing procedure to simply isolate the 0.1% Triton X-100 insoluble fraction of a small volume of positive blood culture broth by centrifugation. The resulting pellet was spread directly onto the MALDI-TOF MS plate for identification in duplicate. A score of ≥ 1.5 with the same identification among the top 3 scores for at least 1 of the 2 duplicate samples allowed their rapid method to identify 80.5% of 632 monomicrobial cultures with a 99.4% accuracy. Overall, 90.5%, 75.6%, 70.6%, and 72.7%, of gram-negatives; gram-positives; *Staphylococcus pneumoniae,* specifically; and nonfermentative gram-negative bacilli were identified to the species level.

MALDI-TOF MS–positive blood culture broth identification consistently struggles to accurately identify polymicrobial blood stream infections.[50] For example, one study of 49 polymicrobial blood stream infections correctly identified 2, 1, or no bacteria in 4.1%, 73.5%, and 22.4% of cases, respectively.[42] Hariu and colleagues[51] spiked blood culture bottles with defined ratios of gram-positive and gram-negative bacteria and found that the MALDI-TOF MS Biotyper was able to identity both organisms when the ratio of both organisms was between 1:3 and 1:1.

Specifically, a version of the MBT Sepsityper module software detects polymicrobial infections processed with the MALDI-TOF MS Sepsityper kit. It currently can identify a maximum of 2 organisms, providing a double identification result to suggest a mixed blood culture. Scohy and colleagues[52] evaluated the software with 143 polymicrobial blood culture bottles containing between 2 and 5 organisms per bottle. The software correctly identified 2 organisms in only 34% of bottles, a single organism in 55% of bottles, no organism in 11% of bottles, and erroneously reported 14 organisms that did not grow in culture.

Identifying yeast directly from positive blood cultures is more challenging than bacteria. Various methods have been tried to improve accurate identification, including additional wash steps during organism purification, increased sample application to MS target plates, and lowering acceptable score cutoffs.[49,53–55] Vecchione and colleagues[49] used a combination of serum separator tubes, sodium dodecyl sulfate treatment for blood cell lysis, and sterile water wash steps to correctly identify more than 50% of yeast with a cutoff of ≥ 1.7, and 87% using a cutoff of ≥ 1.3 with multiple consecutive matches with the same species among the spectra match list. MALDI-TOF MS also can detect biomarkers like dihexasaccharide directly from human serum that may assist in faster and cheaper identification of invasive candidiasis, aspergillosis, and mucormycosis.[56] Further research is needed to evaluate the clinical performance of this assay.

RAPID URINE MATRIX-ASSISTED LASER DESORPTION/IONIZATION TIME-OF-FLIGHT MASS SPECTROMETRY

Urine cultures are one of the highest-volume tests in CMLs. Conventional methodology requires 18 to 48 hours to culture potential pathogens, which can be identified using MALDI-TOF MS, and an additional 24 hours for AST; as such, faster diagnostics would be helpful.[57] Urinary tract infections (UTIs) are typically monomicrobial and contain relatively high organism burden; thus, recent studies focus on purifying microorganisms from urine samples, then using MALDI-TOF MS to identify the potential pathogens. Organism purification techniques vary greatly, and many require substantial hands-on time, including incubations, centrifugation, filtration, diafiltration, lysis, and wash steps.[58–60] Furthermore, some studies suggest protein extraction[61] or ultrasonification may enhance organism identification.[62]

Because sample processing can be time-consuming, many methods recommend using urinalysis or flow cytometry[63–68] to prescreen for samples that are likely to be positive. Samples with $\geq 10^5$ colony-forming units (cfu)/mL to $\geq 5 \times 10^6$ cfu/mL[64,65,67,69] have improved performance and likely represent most patients with true UTI. Recovery of bacteria from urine samples has been variably reported to be compromised by high epithelial and white blood cell numbers,[65,66] which may reflect not yet optimized bacterial isolation procedures.

Most published studies consistently find that bacteria purified directly from urine produce different spectra compared with organisms cultured on solid media[65,70] with associated lower organism identification scores. One notable difference in spectra is the presence of human-derived antimicrobial peptides called α-defensins. These peptides produce 3 strong peaks of approximately 3440 Da, which can hinder database matching.[70] One study changed Bruker's spectra library matching range from 3000 to 15,000 Da to 4000 to 16,000 Da to remove noise from α-defensins, but saw only mild improvement in organism identification. This led Pinault and colleagues[65] to develop a direct-from-urine specific MALDI-TOF MS database (Urinf) using 1000 monomicrobial urine cultures. They then prospectively compared MALDI-TOF MS identification directly from urine samples using Urinf and the standard database,[65] finding 90% versus 50% correct identifications using a cutoff score of ≥ 1.9. Gram-negative bacteria had a higher identification rate than gram-positive bacteria at 90% and 72%, respectively, with inability to identify *Staphylococcus epidermidis*, an infrequent uropathogen, with either database.

Once a potential pathogen has been purified from urine and identified by MALDI-TOF MS, the remaining organism pellet can be used to immediately set up antimicrobial susceptibility testing, including MALDI-TOF MS AST methods described previously, such as carbapenemase detection.[64]

Pathogen identification directly from urine cultures may fulfill an important need, but there are several challenges to address. Many published methods require large volumes of urine, with several requiring ≥ 10 mL, which can be problematic particularly for pediatric populations.[58,64,66] Methods like flow cytometry to prescreen urine samples for suitability are themselves complicated, although simple methods like Bacterioscan for bacterial enumeration in combination with traditional urinalysis may provide sufficient delineation. MALDI-TOF MS may also be useful to identify antigens for pathogens not traditionally diagnosed with urine samples such as syphilis.[71]

SUMMARY

As this review highlights, the utility of MALDI-TOF MS in the CML now extends well beyond organism identification. Even within the realm of organism identification, MALDI-TOF MS is being applied to new areas such as mycobacteriology and mycology. Although these methods are still not commonplace, improvements in database development and workflow make its widespread use for identification of these organisms imminent. In some ways, MALDI-TOF MS has created a problem in that it has accelerated the time frame for organism identification beyond what can be achieved with AST. The new methods discussed herein may help solve this problem by producing definitive AST results in a time frame comparable to organism identification.

Last, MALDI-TOF MS methods for direct identification from clinical specimens such as blood culture bottles and urine specimens have now been developed. Some studies suggest that MALDI-TOF MS may prove higher yield than molecular methods, whereas others have used a combined approach in an effort to control cost and supplement deficiencies in MALDI-TOF MS identification of gram-positive organisms from positive blood cultures.[47,50]

Given these promising applications, it is clear that the MALDI-TOF MS revolution in clinical microbiology is not over and will continue to improve our ability to diagnose infectious diseases.

REFERENCES

1. Mather CA, Rivera SF, Butler-Wu SM. Comparison of the Bruker Biotyper and Vitek MS matrix-assisted laser desorption ionization-time of flight mass spectrometry systems for identification of mycobacteria using simplified protein extraction protocols. J Clin Microbiol 2014;52(1):130–8.
2. Rodriguez-Temporal D, Perez-Risco D, Struzka EA, et al. Evaluation of two protein extraction protocols based on freezing and mechanical disruption for identifying nontuberculous mycobacteria by matrix-assisted laser desorption ionization-time of flight mass spectrometry from liquid and solid cultures. J Clin Microbiol 2018; 56(4) [pii:e01548-17].
3. Luo L, Cao W, Chen W, et al. Evaluation of the VITEK MS knowledge base version 3.0 for the identification of clinically relevant *Mycobacterium* species. Emerg Microbes Infect 2018;7(1):114.
4. Body BA, Beard MA, Slechta ES, et al. Evaluation of the Vitek MS v3.0 matrix-assisted laser desorption ionization-time of flight mass spectrometry system for identification of *Mycobacterium* and *Nocardia* species. J Clin Microbiol 2018; 56(6) [pii:e00237-18].
5. Alcaide F, Amlerova J, Bou G, et al. How to: identify non-tuberculous *Mycobacterium* species using MALDI-TOF mass spectrometry. Clin Microbiol Infect 2018;24(6):599–603.

6. Yan Q, Karau MJ, Greenwood-Quaintance KE, et al. Comparison of diagnostic accuracy of periprosthetic tissue culture in blood culture bottles to that of prosthesis sonication fluid culture for diagnosis of prosthetic joint infection (PJI) by use of bayesian latent class modeling and IDSA PJI criteria for classification. J Clin Microbiol 2018;56(6) [pii:e00319-18].

7. Leyer C, Gregorowicz G, Mougari F, et al. Comparison of saramis 4.12 and IVD 3.0 Vitek MS matrix-assisted laser desorption ionization-time of flight mass spectrometry for identification of mycobacteria from solid and liquid culture media. J Clin Microbiol 2017;55(7):2045–54.

8. Wilen CB, McMullen AR, Burnham CA. Comparison of sample preparation methods, instrumentation platforms, and contemporary commercial databases for identification of clinically relevant mycobacteria by matrix-assisted laser desorption ionization-time of flight mass spectrometry. J Clin Microbiol 2015; 53(7):2308–15.

9. Dupont D, Normand AC, Persat F, et al. Comparison of matrix-assisted laser desorption ionization time of flight mass spectrometry (MALDI-TOF MS) systems for the identification of moulds in the routine microbiology laboratory. Clin Microbiol Infect 2019;25(7):892–7.

10. Stein M, Tran V, Nichol KA, et al. Evaluation of three MALDI-TOF mass spectrometry libraries for the identification of filamentous fungi in three clinical microbiology laboratories in Manitoba, Canada. Mycoses 2018;61(10):743–53.

11. Rychert J, Slechta ES, Barker AP, et al. Multicenter evaluation of the Vitek MS v3.0 system for the identification of filamentous fungi. J Clin Microbiol 2018;56(2) [pii: e01353-17].

12. Normand AC, Cassagne C, Gautier M, et al. Decision criteria for MALDI-TOF MS-based identification of filamentous fungi using commercial and in-house reference databases. BMC Microbiol 2017;17(1):25.

13. Hrabak J, Chudackova E, Walkova R. Matrix-assisted laser desorption ionization-time of flight (maldi-tof) mass spectrometry for detection of antibiotic resistance mechanisms: from research to routine diagnosis. Clin Microbiol Rev 2013;26(1): 103–14.

14. Rhoads DD, Wang H, Karichu J, et al. The presence of a single MALDI-TOF mass spectral peak predicts methicillin resistance in staphylococci. Diagn Microbiol Infect Dis 2016;86(3):257–61.

15. Asakura K, Azechi T, Sasano H, et al. Rapid and easy detection of low-level resistance to vancomycin in methicillin-resistant *Staphylococcus aureus* by matrix-assisted laser desorption ionization time-of-flight mass spectrometry. PLoS One 2018;13(3):e0194212.

16. Lange C, Schubert S, Jung J, et al. Quantitative matrix-assisted laser desorption ionization-time of flight mass spectrometry for rapid resistance detection. J Clin Microbiol 2014;52(12):4155–62.

17. Van Driessche L, Bokma J, Gille L, et al. Rapid detection of tetracycline resistance in bovine Pasteurella multocida isolates by MALDI Biotyper antibiotic susceptibility test rapid assay (MBT-ASTRA). Sci Rep 2018;8(1):13599.

18. Justesen US, Acar Z, Sydenham TV, et al. Antimicrobial susceptibility testing of *Bacteroides fragilis* using the MALDI Biotyper antibiotic susceptibility test rapid assay (MBT-ASTRA). Anaerobe 2018;54:236–9.

19. Jung JS, Eberl T, Sparbier K, et al. Rapid detection of antibiotic resistance based on mass spectrometry and stable isotopes. Eur J Clin Microbiol Infect Dis 2014; 33(6):949–55.

20. Sparbier K, Lange C, Jung J, et al. MALDI biotyper-based rapid resistance detection by stable-isotope labeling. J Clin Microbiol 2013;51(11):3741–8.
21. Idelevich EA, Sparbier K, Kostrzewa M, et al. Rapid detection of antibiotic resistance by MALDI-TOF mass spectrometry using a novel direct-on-target microdroplet growth assay. Clin Microbiol Infect 2018;24(7):738–43.
22. Li M, Liu M, Song Q, et al. Rapid antimicrobial susceptibility testing by matrix-assisted laser desorption ionization-time of flight mass spectrometry using a qualitative method in *Acinetobacter baumannii* complex. J Microbiol Methods 2018;153:60–5.
23. Idelevich EA, Storck LM, Sparbier K, et al. Rapid direct susceptibility testing from positive blood cultures by the matrix-assisted laser desorption ionization-time of flight mass spectrometry-based direct-on-target microdroplet growth assay. J Clin Microbiol 2018;56(10) [pii:e00913-18].
24. Marinach C, Alanio A, Palous M, et al. MALDI-TOF MS-based drug susceptibility testing of pathogens: the example of *Candida albicans* and fluconazole. Proteomics 2009;9(20):4627–31.
25. Vella A, De Carolis E, Vaccaro L, et al. Rapid antifungal susceptibility testing by matrix-assisted laser desorption ionization-time of flight mass spectrometry analysis. J Clin Microbiol 2013;51(9):2964–9.
26. Paul S, Singh P, A S S, et al. Rapid detection of fluconazole resistance in *Candida tropicalis* by MALDI-TOF MS. Med Mycol 2018;56(2):234–41.
27. Saracli MA, Fothergill AW, Sutton DA, et al. Detection of triazole resistance among *Candida* species by matrix-assisted laser desorption/ionization-time of flight mass spectrometry (MALDI-TOF MS). Med Mycol 2015;53(7):736–42.
28. De Carolis E, Vella A, Florio AR, et al. Use of matrix-assisted laser desorption ionization-time of flight mass spectrometry for caspofungin susceptibility testing of *Candida* and *Aspergillus* species. J Clin Microbiol 2012;50(7):2479–83.
29. Gitman MR, McTaggart L, Spinato J, et al. Antifungal susceptibility testing of aspergillus spp. by using a composite correlation index (CCI)-based matrix-assisted laser desorption ionization-time of flight mass spectrometry method appears to not offer benefit over traditional broth microdilution testing. J Clin Microbiol 2017;55(7):2030–4.
30. Vatanshenassan M, Boekhout T, Lass-Florl C, et al. Proof of concept for MBT AS-TRA, a rapid matrix-assisted laser desorption ionization-time of flight mass spectrometry (MALDI-TOF MS)-based method to detect Caspofungin resistance in *Candida albicans* and *Candida glabrata*. J Clin Microbiol 2018;56(9) [pii: e00420-18].
31. Ceyssens PJ, Soetaert K, Timke M, et al. Matrix-assisted laser desorption ionization-time of flight mass spectrometry for combined species identification and drug sensitivity testing in mycobacteria. J Clin Microbiol 2017;55(2):624–34.
32. Klein S, Zimmermann S, Kohler C, et al. Integration of matrix-assisted laser desorption/ionization time-of-flight mass spectrometry in blood culture diagnostics: a fast and effective approach. J Med Microbiol 2012;61(Pt 3):323–31.
33. Drancourt M. Detection of microorganisms in blood specimens using matrix-assisted laser desorption ionization time-of-flight mass spectrometry: a review. Clin Microbiol Infect 2010;16(11):1620–5.
34. Christner M, Rohde H, Wolters M, et al. Rapid identification of bacteria from positive blood culture bottles by use of matrix-assisted laser desorption-ionization time of flight mass spectrometry fingerprinting. J Clin Microbiol 2010;48(5):1584–91.

35. Idelevich EA, Schule I, Grunastel B, et al. Rapid identification of microorganisms from positive blood cultures by MALDI-TOF mass spectrometry subsequent to very short-term incubation on solid medium. Clin Microbiol Infect 2014;20(10): 1001–6.

36. Verroken A, Defourny L, Lechgar L, et al. Reducing time to identification of positive blood cultures with MALDI-TOF MS analysis after a 5-h subculture. Eur J Clin Microbiol Infect Dis 2015;34(2):405–13.

37. Verhoeven PO, Haddar CH, Rigaill J, et al. Comparison of the fully automated FilmArray BCID assay to a 4-hour culture test coupled to mass spectrometry for day 0 identification of microorganisms in positive blood cultures. Biomed Research International 2018;2018:7013470.

38. Shannon S, Kronemann D, Patel R, et al. Routine use of MALDI-TOF MS for anaerobic bacterial identification in clinical microbiology. Anaerobe 2018;54:191–6.

39. Altun O, Botero-Kleiven S, Carlsson S, et al. Rapid identification of bacteria from positive blood culture bottles by MALDI-TOF MS following short-term incubation on solid media. J Med Microbiol 2015;64(11):1346–52.

40. Halavaara M, Nevalainen A, Martelius T, et al. Impact of short-incubation MALDI-TOF MS on empiric antibiotic therapy in bloodstream infections caused by Pseudomonas aeruginosa, Enterococcus spp. and AmpC-producing Enterobacteriaceae. Diagn Microbiol Infect Dis 2019;94(1):1–6.

41. Morgenthaler NG, Kostrzewa M. Rapid identification of pathogens in positive blood culture of patients with sepsis: review and meta-analysis of the performance of the sepsityper kit. Int J Microbiol 2015;2015:827416.

42. Simon L, Ughetto E, Gaudart A, et al. Direct identification of 80 percent of bacteria from blood culture bottles by matrix-assisted laser desorption ionization-time of flight mass spectrometry using a 10-minute extraction protocol. J Clin Microbiol 2019;57(2) [pii:e01278-18].

43. Wu S, Xu J, Qiu C, et al. Direct antimicrobial susceptibility tests of bacteria and yeasts from positive blood cultures by using serum separator gel tubes and MALDI-TOF MS. J Microbiol Methods 2019;157:16–20.

44. Fiori B, D'Inzeo T, Di Florio V, et al. Performance of two resin-containing blood culture media in detection of bloodstream infections and in direct matrix-assisted laser desorption ionization-time of flight mass spectrometry (MALDI-TOF MS) broth assays for isolate identification: clinical comparison of the BacT/Alert Plus and Bactec Plus systems. J Clin Microbiol 2014;52(10):3558–67.

45. Azrad M, Keness Y, Nitzan O, et al. Cheap and rapid in-house method for direct identification of positive blood cultures by MALDI-TOF MS technology. BMC Infect Dis 2019;19(1):72.

46. Zhou M, Yang Q, Kudinha T, et al. An improved in-house MALDI-TOF MS protocol for direct cost-effective identification of pathogens from blood cultures. Front Microbiol 2017;8:1824.

47. Arroyo MA, Denys GA. Parallel evaluation of the MALDI sepsityper and verigene BC-GN assays for rapid identification of gram-negative Bacilli from positive blood cultures. J Clin Microbiol 2017;55(9):2708–18.

48. Barnini S, Ghelardi E, Brucculeri V, et al. Rapid and reliable identification of gram-negative bacteria and gram-positive cocci by deposition of bacteria harvested from blood cultures onto the MALDI-TOF plate. BMC Microbiol 2015;15:124.

49. Vecchione A, Florio W, Celandroni F, et al. A rapid procedure for identification and antifungal susceptibility testing of yeasts from positive blood cultures. Front Microbiol 2018;9:2400.

50. Fiori B, D'Inzeo T, Giaquinto A, et al. Optimized use of the MALDI BioTyper system and the FilmArray BCID panel for direct identification of microbial pathogens from positive blood cultures. J Clin Microbiol 2016;54(3):576–84.

51. Hariu M, Watanabe Y, Oikawa N, et al. Usefulness of matrix-assisted laser desorption ionization time-of-flight mass spectrometry to identify pathogens, including polymicrobial samples, directly from blood culture broths. Infect Drug Resist 2017;10:115–20.

52. Scohy A, Noel A, Boeras A, et al. Evaluation of the Bruker(R) MBT Sepsityper IVD module for the identification of polymicrobial blood cultures with MALDI-TOF MS. Eur J Clin Microbiol Infect Dis 2018;37(11):2145–52.

53. Idelevich EA, Grunewald CM, Wullenweber J, et al. Rapid identification and susceptibility testing of *Candida* spp. from positive blood cultures by combination of direct MALDI-TOF mass spectrometry and direct inoculation of Vitek 2. PloS one 2014;9(12):e114834.

54. Spanu T, Posteraro B, Fiori B, et al. Direct MALDI-TOF mass spectrometry assay of blood culture broths for rapid identification of *Candida* species causing bloodstream infections: an observational study in two large microbiology laboratories. J Clin Microbiol 2012;50(1):176–9.

55. Yan Y, He Y, Maier T, et al. Improved identification of yeast species directly from positive blood culture media by combining Sepsityper specimen processing and Microflex analysis with the matrix-assisted laser desorption ionization Biotyper system. J Clin Microbiol 2011;49(7):2528–32.

56. Mery A, Sendid B, Francois N, et al. Application of mass spectrometry technology to early diagnosis of invasive fungal infections. J Clin Microbiol 2016;54(11):2786–97.

57. Yan Y, Meng S, Bian D, et al. Comparative evaluation of Bruker Biotyper and BD Phoenix systems for identification of bacterial pathogens associated with urinary tract infections. J Clin Microbiol 2011;49(11):3936–9.

58. Demarco ML, Burnham CA. Diafiltration MALDI-TOF mass spectrometry method for culture-independent detection and identification of pathogens directly from urine specimens. Am J Clin Pathol 2014;141(2):204–12.

59. Haiko J, Savolainen LE, Hilla R, et al. Identification of urinary tract pathogens after 3-hours urine culture by MALDI-TOF mass spectrometry. J Microbiol Methods 2016;129:81–4.

60. Veron L, Mailler S, Girard V, et al. Rapid urine preparation prior to identification of uropathogens by MALDI-TOF MS. Eur J Clin Microbiol Infect Dis 2015;34(9):1787–95.

61. Ferreira L, Sanchez-Juanes F, Gonzalez-Avila M, et al. Direct identification of urinary tract pathogens from urine samples by matrix-assisted laser desorption ionization-time of flight mass spectrometry. J Clin Microbiol 2010;48(6):2110–5.

62. Kitagawa K, Shigemura K, Onuma KI, et al. Improved bacterial identification directly from urine samples with matrix-assisted laser desorption/ionization time-of-flight mass spectrometry. J Clin Lab Anal 2018;32(3).

63. Huang B, Zhang L, Zhang W, et al. Direct detection and identification of bacterial pathogens from urine with optimized specimen processing and enhanced testing algorithm. J Clin Microbiol 2017;55(5):1488–95.

64. Oviano M, Ramirez CL, Barbeyto LP, et al. Rapid direct detection of carbapenemase-producing Enterobacteriaceae in clinical urine samples by MALDI-TOF MS analysis. J Antimicrob Chemother 2017;72(5):1350–4.

65. Pinault L, Chabrière E, Raoult D, et al. Direct identification of pathogens in urine by use of a specific matrix-assisted laser desorption ionization-time of flight spectrum database. J Clin Microbiol 2019;57(4) [pii:e01678-18].

66. Zboromyrska Y, Bosch J, Aramburu J, et al. A multicentre study investigating parameters which influence direct bacterial identification from urine. PloS one 2018; 13(12):e0207822.

67. Zboromyrska Y, Rubio E, Alejo I, et al. Development of a new protocol for rapid bacterial identification and susceptibility testing directly from urine samples. Clin Microbiol Infect 2016;22(6):561.e1-6.

68. Inigo M, Coello A, Fernandez-Rivas G, et al. Direct identification of urinary tract pathogens from urine samples, combining urine screening methods and matrix-assisted laser desorption ionization-time of flight mass spectrometry. J Clin Microbiol 2016;54(4):988–93.

69. Wang XH, Zhang G, Fan YY, et al. Direct identification of bacteria causing urinary tract infections by combining matrix-assisted laser desorption ionization-time of flight mass spectrometry with UF-1000i urine flow cytometry. J Microbiol Methods 2013;92(3):231–5.

70. Kohling HL, Bittner A, Muller KD, et al. Direct identification of bacteria in urine samples by matrix-assisted laser desorption/ionization time-of-flight mass spectrometry and relevance of defensins as interfering factors. J Med Microbiol 2012;61(Pt 3):339–44.

71. Osbak KK, Van Raemdonck GA, Dom M, et al. Candidate *Treponema pallidum* biomarkers uncovered in urine from individuals with syphilis using mass spectrometry. Future Microbiol 2018;13:1497–510.

Next-Generation Sequencing in Clinical Microbiology: Are We There Yet?

Stephanie L. Mitchell, PhD, D(ABMM)[a],
Patricia J. Simner, PhD, D(ABMM)[b],*

KEYWORDS

- Next-generation sequencing (NGS) • Whole-genome sequencing (WGS)
- Targeted next-generation sequencing (tNGS)
- Metagenomics next-generations sequencing (mNGS) • Clinical microbiology
- Infectious disease

KEY POINTS

- The 3 main applications of next-generation sequencing in clinical microbiology laboratories include (1) whole-genome sequencing (WGS), (2) targeted next-generation sequencing (tNGS), and (3) metagenomics next-generation sequencing.
- WGS is becoming commonplace in public health laboratories, aiding in the rapid identification and tracking of infectious disease outbreaks alongside detection of emerging resistance and surveillance.
- tNGS has been underutilized in clinical microbiology; however, the development of new enrichment methods will allow for broad pathogen detection combined with high sensitivity. tNGS may become a more accessible assay in the future.
- Metagenomic next-generation sequencing has emerged as a promising single, universal pathogen detection (ie, bacteria, fungi, parasites, viruses) method for infectious diseases diagnostics performed directly from clinical specimens. Laboratory-developed tests are now being offered as billable tests; understanding the limitations of these nonstandardized and expensive tests is imperative for appropriate test utilization and result interpretation.

Continued

Disclosure Statement: P.J. Simner reports grants and personal fees from Accelerate Diagnostics, grants from BD Diagnostics, Inc, grants from bioMerieux, Inc, grants from Check-Points Diagnostics, BV, grants from Hardy Diagnostics, personal fees from Roche Diagnostics, personal fees from Opgen Inc, personal fees from CosmosID, outside the submitted work. P.J. Simner reports travel funds from Oxford Nanopore Technologies. S.L. Mitchell is a member of GenMark Diagnostic's Scientific Advisory Board.
[a] Department of Pathology, UPMC Children's Hospital of Pittsburgh, University of Pittsburgh School of Medicine, 4401 Penn Avenue, Main Hospital, Floor B, #269, Pittsburgh, PA 15224, USA; [b] Division of Medical Microbiology, Department of Pathology, Johns Hopkins University School of Medicine, Meyer B1-193, 600 North Wolfe Street, Baltimore, MD 21287-7093, USA
* Corresponding author.
E-mail address: psimner1@jhmi.edu

Continued

- Over the next 5 to 10 years, more mid- to large-size laboratories are likely to be seen implementing next-generation sequencing as the cost of sequencing continues to decrease and as the diagnostics and informatics become more automated with shorter turn-around times.

INTRODUCTION

Next-generation sequencing (NGS) is a method that allows for high-throughput, massively parallel sequencing of thousands to billions of DNA fragments independently and simultaneously.[1] Over the last 5 years, NGS applications have been transitioning from research tools into diagnostic methods and are becoming more commonplace in clinical microbiology laboratories. These applications include (1) whole-genome sequencing (WGS), (2) targeted next-generation sequencing (tNGS) methods, and (3) metagenomic next-generation sequencing (mNGS); all of which are defined (**Fig. 1**, **Table 1**) and described in further detail herein. These applications can be further adapted to answer specific diagnostic questions in regard to strain typing in outbreak investigations,[2,3] or predicting susceptibility to antimicrobial agents[4] or pan-pathogen detection directly from specimens,[5] to name a few.

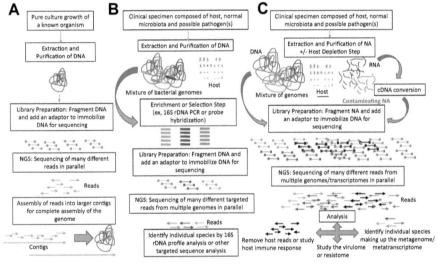

Fig. 1. The different applications of NGS in clinical microbiology laboratories. (*A*) WGS of a pure organism from cultured growth. (*B*) tNGS directly from specimen (example: 16S rDNA from a clinical specimen for bacterial profiling). (*C*) mNGS from clinical specimens. The nucleic acid (NA) composition of the specimens includes host (*black*), microbiome and pathogen detection (*blue, green,* and *red*), and last, the inadvertent introduction of contaminating nucleic acid (*orange*). Analysis of reads generally involves removing host nucleic acid from microbial NA. The microbial reads are analyzed to identify the composition and abundance of reads of organisms present or to study the resistome or virulome. The study of RNA can allow for transcriptome-based analysis to identify organisms that are transcriptionally active. cDNA, complementary DNA. (*Modified from* Simner PJ, Miller S, Carroll KC. Understanding the promises and hurdles of metagenomic next-generation sequencing as a diagnostic tool for infectious diseases. Clin Infect Dis 2018;66(5):780; with permission.)

Table 1
Glossary of terms used in next-generation sequencing applications

Term (Abbreviation)	Definition
Metagenomic Next-Generation Sequencing (mNGS; also known as agnostic or unbiased NGS)	Allows for pan-nucleic acid detection directly from patient specimens. All nucleic acid within a specimen is extracted and sequenced in parallel, resulting in sequencing of both host and microbial reads. This approach can include both a DNA and an RNA method. The RNA method may be referred to specifically as metatranscriptomic NGS.[1,37,65]
Whole-genome sequencing (WGS)	Sequencing and assembly of a microbial genome. WGS can be applied to pure culture growth of a microbial organism (bacterial) or directly from specimen (viral).
Targeted next-generation sequencing (tNGS)	Uses a selection process to enrich for specific targets before sequencing. Examples include 16S rDNA bacterial profiling or PCR amplification of other specified targets followed by NGS.
Next-generation sequencing (NGS)	High-throughput, massively parallel sequencing of thousands up to billions of DNA fragments independently and simultaneously.
Read	The basic element produced by DNA sequencing. Reads are composed of a series of sequential bases making up the DNA fragment, which can vary in size from small reads (50–700 bp) to long reads (1000–10,000s bp) depending on the sequencing technology.[65]
Microbiome	Sequencing analysis of a community of microbes in a specimen. Microbiome analysis can be targeted to a specific microbial group (ie, 16S rDNA bacterial profiling) or unbiased using a metagenomics approach.
Resistome	All AMR genes in a given organism or microbiome.
Virulome	All genes that contribute to virulence in a given organism or microbiome.
Cell-free DNA (cfDNA)	Small, unencapsulated, DNA fragments that are debris of the genomes of dead, lysed microorganisms circulating in specimens. mNGS or tNGS of cfDNA can be performed directly from clinical specimens, which may allow for diagnosis of infections from distant sites (ie, pneumonia where DNA is shed into blood from the source).[53]
Secod-generation NGS platform	NGS platform that generates short-read sequences (50–700 bp), such as Illumina and Ion Torrent.
Third-generation NGS platform	NGS platform that generates long-read sequences (1000–10,000s bp) at the single-molecule level, such as PacBio and Oxford Nanopore.
Bioinformatics	Conceptualizes biology in terms of macromolecules and then applies informatics techniques (applied math, computer science, and statistics) to understand and organize the information associated with these molecules on a large scale.[66]
Bioinformatics pipeline	Bioinformatics algorithms executed in a predefined sequence to process NGS data. A pipeline progressively shepherds and processes massive sequence data and their associated metadata through a series of transformations using multiple software components, databases, and operation environments.[67]

Whole-Genome Sequencing

WGS is the sequencing and assembly of a microbial genome. To date, the most common use of WGS is for simultaneous identification, typing, and/or antimicrobial susceptibility prediction for microbial pathogens. Methods for performing WGS may differ depending on what pathogen is in question. WGS of viral genomes does not require culture or isolation of the virus and is typically performed directly from patient samples. Alternatively, for bacteria, the presence of other bacteria in clinical specimens that are either clinically insignificant, such as normal skin flora, or represent polymicrobial infections, may confound WGS results, especially when attempting to predict resistance profiles with mechanisms carried on plasmids or other mobile elements. Therefore, current WGS of bacterial pathogens requires culture and isolation of the organism before nucleic acid extraction and sequencing preparations. This has obvious limitations when the organism is difficult to culture or uncultivable. Although this approach also holds true for mycobacterial organisms, methods for mycobacterial WGS directly from clinical isolates have been developed.[6–8]

WGS has proven especially useful in hospital and public health epidemiologic studies by identifying and tracking outbreaks. For example, WGS was capable of detecting and monitoring transmission of a CTX-M-15–producing *Klebsiella pneumoniae* clone and colistin-resistant carbapenemase-producing *K pneumoniae* isolate, thus directing infection control interventions and preventing further spread of these multidrug-resistant organisms.[2,3] WGS of Adenovirus genomes isolated from patients in a neonatal intensive care unit helped identify and contain an outbreak and provided better resolution than typing of the hexon gene by Sanger sequencing.[9] Furthermore, through WGS of Adenovirus-positive environmental samples, the exposure and route of infection were determined and resulted in a change in infection control practices.[9] Beyond hospital epidemiology and infection control applications, WGS has supported public health initiatives to rapidly detect, respond to, and halt the spread of pathogens.[10–12] WGS has allowed enhanced interrogation of potential outbreak strains and their relatedness, leading to better understanding of routes of exposure and transmission.[13,14]

In addition to identification and tracking of outbreaks, WGS provides potentially untapped information regarding pathogen virulence and detection of novel mechanisms of resistance. Virulence can be studied via identification of virulence factor genes, which is currently neither detected by clinical laboratories nor used in patient treatment and management decisions. For example, 1 study highlighted its potential utility for detecting and typing select virulence genes, such as *spa* and PVL toxins, in *Staphylococcus aureus*.[15] In addition, WGS can provide early detection of novel mechanisms of resistance, which traditional molecular detection methods, such as polymerase chain reaction (PCR) of a specific gene or locus, may miss. One example of the value of WGS in detecting novel mutations is the discovery of a synonymous mutation in *Rv3792* in *Mycobacterium tuberculosis* that resulted in elevated ethambutol MICs by increasing expression of the downstream *embC* gene.[16]

Similar to the applications mentioned above, WGS may provide a more detailed analysis of viral pathogens and their resistance as well. Although genetic detection of resistance via Sanger sequencing is currently available for some viral pathogens, mainly human immunodeficiency virus (HIV) and cytomegalovirus (CMV), investigation into use of WGS is being explored. One study using a genome-wide association study for HIV was able to accurately detect 5 genetic associations that lead to amino acid changes known to confer drug resistance.[17] One of the largest potential advantages to a viral WGS approach is the ability to detect resistant subpopulations, which Sanger cannot. One study demonstrated that WGS of HIV increased sensitivity for detecting low-frequency drug-resistant mutations in HIV-1.[18]

One of the most exciting potential applications of WGS is its ability to predict antimicrobial resistance (AMR), which may provide preliminary results more quickly than traditional phenotypic methods. Many published reports have shown promise of using WGS as a molecular antimicrobial testing method for detecting resistance in a variety of bacteria, demonstrating high correlation between resistance genotypes and phenotypic results. One study demonstrated a 97.8% specificity and 99.6% sensitivity for 76 *Escherichia coli* strains tested against 15 antimicrobials.[19] Similar sensitivity and specificity ($\geq$90%) were observed in other studies testing *K pneumoniae*,[20,21] *Pseudomonas aeruginosa*,[22] *S aureus*,[23] and *Neisseria gonorrhoeae*,[24] among others. More recently, machine learning models have been applied based on WGS to predict minimum inhibitory concentrations of antibiotics with an average accuracy of 95% for nontyphoidal *Salmonella*[25] and 92% for *K pneumoniae*.[21]

Given the prolonged time required for phenotypic susceptibility testing for *M tuberculosis*, there is considerable interest in use of WGS for predicting *M tuberculosis* complex susceptibility. Currently, PCR and sequencing of known resistance mutations are being offered by clinical and public health laboratories, providing primary results to aid in treatment decisions and patient management. However, a recent publication evaluated the use of WGS compared with line probes and phenotypic aspartate aminotransferase (AST). WGS-based predictions showed an overall concordance of 99.3%, with a sensitivity of 97.6% and specificity of 99.5%. However, of note, 3.6% of isolates failed to sequence and 10% had insufficient sequence data to make AST predictions.[26] Nevertheless, 1 distinct advantage was that 5.2% of cases had indeterminate WGS resistance predictions due to novel, previously uncharacterized mutations.[26] Other studies assessing WGS have shown similar results[6–8] or slightly lower concordance of 89.2% and 82.6%, respectively.[27,28]

Although the results from WGS-based susceptibility predictions are encouraging, several challenges remain. Published data have focused on the detection of known resistance genes and mutations, but have not necessarily demonstrated the ability of WGS to detect or predict susceptibility. In addition, WGS may be inadequate in detecting mechanisms of resistance that have not been fully elucidated, such as alterations of cell membrane permeability, efflux pump changes, and variations in lipopolysaccharide.[29] Although detection of loss-of-function mutations or acquisition of enzymes known to cleave certain drugs is relatively easy to interpret, mutations in coding or noncoding regions of the genome that alter the structure, dynamics, and substrate specificity of proteins, enzymes, and cell wall components are more challenging to interpret. Without complete knowledge of the impact of a mutation, predicting effects on susceptibility can be problematic and is a noteworthy limitation of WGS.[29] Furthermore, differences have been observed when comparing analysis methods and databases for determining resistance, making it critical to assess pipelines to ensure proper susceptible/resistance designations.[23,30,31]

Most studies to date have applied second-generation sequencing platforms, whereby turnaround times (TAT) are similar to, if not longer than, standard phenotypic AST results.[19,28,32–34] A recent study by Tamma and colleagues[4] applied third-generation Oxford Nanopore WGS that allows for real-time analysis of reads to predict phenotypic AST results within 14 hours of isolation of carbapenem-resistant *K pneumoniae* clinical isolates. Using this approach, they demonstrated the potential to reduce time to effective antibiotic therapy for infections caused by these MDROs by a minimum of 20 hours compared with traditional phenotypic AST. However, until the breadth of mutations, genes, nongenetic alternations, and the combination of those mechanisms that confer AMR are better understood, phenotypic AST remains critically important to provide susceptibility information used in clinical treatment decisions and continues to be the gold standard for detecting susceptibility and resistance.

Targeted Next-Generation Sequencing

tNGS use a selection process before library preparation and sequencing to enrich for microbial sequences of interest. Enrichment can be achieved by a variety of selection methods, such as PCR amplification (commonly referred to as amplicon sequencing), probe hybridization, and by utilization of CRISPR-Cas9.[35,36] The advantages of tNGS over a metagenomic approach is that it overcomes the "needle in the haystack" dilemma of amplifying low numbers of microbial sequences within highly cellular samples.[37] However, the enrichment process (eg, multiplex PCR for specific genes) may introduce target bias.

For clinical applications of tNGS, the main goal is to identify the microbial pathogen or pathogens in patient samples; however, assays may also target antibiotic resistance genes. The most common enrichment method used to date for clinical applications and microbiome studies is amplification of the 16S ribosomal RNA (rRNA) gene by PCR before NGS.[35,38,39] However, alternative methods for enrichment are also being developed. One such approach was described by Sabat and colleagues,[40] who developed a bacterial tNGS assay that amplified by PCR and sequenced the entire 16S-23S rRNA region in urine samples from patients with suspected urinary tract infection, positive blood cultures, and orthopedic samples. Compared with conventional culture, identification by commercial systems, and 16S Sanger sequencing, the 16S-23S tNGS assay correctly identified pathogens from blood and urine and showed increased detection of bacterial pathogens from orthopedic samples.[40] Although interpretation of 16S data can be challenging and often provides only genus level identifications, the inclusion of the 23S region appears to enhance specificity and sensitivity.

In addition to simplex tNGS assays, larger multiplex panels are being developed. Two assays using a multiplex probe enrichment step for both viral (VirCapSeq-VERT) and bacterial (BacCapSeq) detection in blood and tissue samples have been described.[41,42] Both use a pool of 2 to 4 million probes to select for microbial sequences covering more than 300 bacterial and 200 viral species, respectively, inclusive of AMR markers and virulence determinants for the former.[41,42] These assays showed similar limits of detection when compared with specific singleplex PCRs. VirCapSeq-VERT has been applied clinically, where it was compared with mNGS for determination of the causative agent of fever of unknown origin.[43] Although the same organisms were identified by both methods, VirCapSeq had higher sensitivity compared with the metagenomic method.[43] Not unsurprisingly, the unbiased mNGS approach provided better genome coverage because of the ability to sequence all areas of the genome, whereas VirCapSeq will only sequence genomic areas that are selected by the probes.[43] However, if the goal of the assay is simply to identify a microbial pathogen, complete genome coverage is not necessary, and increased sensitivity provided by a selection process would be preferred.

Although the focus of tNGS appears to be mostly for identification, a tNGS assay using amplicon sequencing to detect CMV viral resistance in clinical samples was shown to be highly sensitive, particularly for minor variants.[44] Although this study highlights the utility of tNGS in detecting well-characterized resistance mechanisms, this approach has similar limitations to WGS for accurately predicting phenotypic suscep-tibility, particularly for bacteria.

Further exploration is clearly needed to define the role of tNGS in clinical diagnostics and relative merits compared with alternative technologies, such as molecular multi-plex panels (see Marc Roger Couturier and Jennifer Dien Bard's article, "Direct-from-Specimen Pathogen Identification: Evolution of Syndromic Panels," in this issue.)

Metagenomic Next-Generation Sequencing

mNGS is a method that allows for pan-nucleic acid detection directly from patient specimens.[1] This approach, unlike tNGS methods, does not selectively amplify spe-cific targets because all nucleic acids in a sample are amplified and sequenced in par-allel, allowing for unbiased detection of all microbial groups (ie, bacterial, viral, parasite, and fungal agents), resistance markers, virulence factors, or even host bio-markers associated with different disease states. This provides the advantage of a hypothesis-free diagnostic directly from patient specimens.

Methodologic variants include DNA and RNA (also known as metatranscriptomics) -based methods that detect intact microbes from the source of infection or cell-free DNA (cfDNA). cfDNA, small nucleic acid fragments from dead, lysed microorganisms filtered into blood or urine, may provide a readout for distant sites of infection (eg, lung during pneumonia). It is important to understand the differences and limitations of these methods. For example, if an RNA-based approach is not included in the mNGS procedure, RNA viruses will not be able to be detected or transcriptome-based analysis will not be able to be applied to study the host immune response. Re-sults from cfDNA will not always reveal the source of infection or the true cause because a high background of detectable microbial cfDNA has been demonstrated in plasma of asymptomatic individuals (60/162 patients: 22%).[45] mNGS methodolo-gies are also complex, multistep processes that currently lack standardization, further complicating result interpretation.[46]

mNGS has proven successful as a diagnostic tool in detecting infections in multiple sites, including the central nervous system,[46–48] bloodstream,[43,45] respiratory,[49] gastrointestinal,[50] prosthetic joint,[51,52] urinary tract,[53] and ocular.[54] Pathogens identi-fied included bacteria,[5,46,47,49,51,52] mycobacteria,[47,55] RNA and DNA viruses,[54,55] yeast and molds,[36,48] and parasites.[48,54] In a few of these cases, large batteries of standard diagnostic tools were unrevealing. mNGS was particularly successful for detection of novel,[56] rare,[5] and atypical causes[57] or in previously treated patients.[53,58]

What additional yield does mNGS provide above standard-of-care testing for pa-tient management, especially for this rather expensive and labor-intensive method? A few recent studies suggest enhanced sensitivity of mNGS compared with standard-of-care diagnostics and are instructive as to the promise of mNGS. A study by Miao and colleagues[55] examined comparative performance on 511 specimens of various sources. A retrospective chart review indicated an overall clinical sensitivity and specificity of 50.7% and 85.7% for mNGS and 35.2% and 89.1% for standard di-agnostics, respectively. mNGS excelled especially for M tuberculosis, viruses, anaer-obes, and fungi. However, the same study also suggested that detection by mNGS is not superior to culture for common bacterial infections, especially when there is no previous antibiotic exposure. Similarly, mNGS of sonicate fluids or synovial fluid from prosthetic joint infection provided an incremental 25% and 18.3% yield in culture-negative cases, respectively.[51,52] Another case series of 94 patients used mNGS to examine cerebrospinal fluid in patients with subacute or chronic meningitis, identifying 2 Taenia solium, 1 HIV-1, and 4 fungal pathogens. One case of subarach-noid neurocysticercosis had eluded diagnosis for a year.[59] This study demonstrated that there is often a large denominator of mostly negative cases or cases with no actionable results.[60] However, occasionally, mNGS is able to identify a previously unknown pathogen and be helpful for patient management.[48,61]

Most initial efforts have focused on pathogen detection. However, mNGS sequence may also be used to strain type predominant pathogen or pathogens or detect AMR and virulence factor genes directly from specimens, when there is sufficient coverage. This is easier for pathogens with smaller genomes, such as viruses. For example, strain typing of Zika virus in the blood linked acquisition in an endemic area due to a subsequent secondary, nonsexual transmission case.[62] Yan and colleagues[63] recently applied the CosmosID bioinformatics platform to query mNGS results positive for staphylococci to detect *mecA*-mediated methicillin resistance with 77.4% sensitivity and 100% specificity. Last, host reads in RNA-based methods can be queried to study the immune response and integrated into the diagnostic algorithm to help assign the significance of microbial reads. Impressively, Langelier and colleagues[64] combined pathogen, microbiome, and host transcriptome analysis in lower-respiratory-tract infections, achieving a negative predictive value of 100%.

Despite these successes, it is imperative to understand the limitations of these methods.

- Most reads sequenced ($\geq$90%) map to *Homo sapiens*.[65] This results in decreased analytical sensitivity for detection of low-burden microbial reads. Host nucleic acid depletion methods have been applied to address this issue.[46,58]
- Microbial reads may reflect colonization (ie, normal microbiota) or infection, or contaminants introduced during specimen collection or extraneous nucleic acid found in reagents (the "kitome") or introduced during laboratory processing (the "labome").[59]
- The LOD will vary based on the methods used and the cellularity of the specimen. Standard-of-care methods and targeted-based approaches (ie, targeted PCR) for the most common pathogens are often more sensitive than mNGS approaches.[65]
- Highly curated databases are required because false-negative or false-positive results may occur.[65]
- The TAT ranges from hours to up to a week (average of 48 hours) from specimen receipt, depending on the sequencing technology, methods, and bioinformatics programs used.
- The cost of sequencing is high whether it is being performed in-house or outsourced. Sequencing in-house requires significant resources for equipment (>$500,000 for the instrument) and reagents (>$100,000 for development to validation). If the test is being outsourced on a case-by-case basis, the average cost per test ranges from $2000 to $3500.
- Reimbursement is unlikely.[61]

Use of Next-Generation Sequencing for Clinical Care: Where Are We at Now?

To date, there are no Food and Drug Administration–cleared NGS-based assays for infectious disease diagnostics. However, many laboratory-developed tests have been established for the different NGS applications. The advantages and disadvantages of these applications are described in **Table 2**. WGS has found current applications especially in the public health sector for epidemiologic investigation and is beginning to transform direct and indirect AST for *M tuberculosis*. tNGS has thus far found limited application for direct specimen analysis for bacteria similar to Sanger sequencing, whereas mNGS has found utility in identifying unsuspected causes in very problematic clinical cases.

Table 2
Advantages and disadvantages of next-generation sequencing applications in clinical microbiology

NGS Application	Advantages	Disadvantages
WGS	• Generates identification and typing information • Predictions of AMR profiles • Discover novel resistance mechanisms • Study virulence factors • Provides entire genome and plasmid sequences • Allows for single nucleotide polymorphism and mutational analysis	• Bacterial WGS requires growth and isolation of pure colony • Cannot accurately predict susceptibility • Some predictions unreliable for certain mechanisms of resistance • Predicted AST profiles must be confirmed by phenotypic AST • Large depth of coverage needed across entire genome (higher sequencing depth and cost)
tNGS	• Determines presence or absence of a pathogen and some known resistance gene/mutations based on target selection • Decreases or eliminates amplification of unwanted human sequences • Highly sensitive • Creation of "syndromic" panels or selection of a group of pathogens commonly tested for specific disease processes • Helpful as an adjunct where slow-growing pathogens are suspected (fungi, AFB) or when patients have previously been exposed to antimicrobials	• Biased (positive selection) • Additional cost for enrichment steps in sample preparation
mNGS	• Unbiased pathogen detection directly from patient specimens • Helpful for the diagnosis of rare, atypical, and novel causes • Helpful as an adjunct where slow-growing pathogens are suspected (fungi, AFB) or when patients have previously been exposed to antimicrobials • Ability to strain type directly from specimens, study virulence, and AMR genes, and evaluate the host immune response • Ability to provide a precision medicine-based approach to diagnosis	• The majority (>90%) of reads are of human origin • TAT is still long and in most cases longer than most standard-of-care methods • Expensive • Reimbursement by insurers or Medicare is unlikely • Complex, multistep processes requiring significant expertise of staff performing testing • Results interpretation can be complex • LOD varies by specimen and methods • Lack of standardization and automation

What Does the Future Hold for Next-Generation Sequencing in Clinical Microbiology Laboratories?

Over the next 5 to 10 years, more mid- to large-size laboratories implementing NGS are likely to be seen as the cost of sequencing continues to decrease and as the diagnostics and informatics become more automated with shorter TAT. Most laboratories will implement WGS as a replacement for pulsed field gel electrophoresis for strain typing and tNGS methods (16S recombinant DNA [rDNA] bacterial profiling) for direct specimen diagnostics as costs become competitive with Sanger sequencing alternatives, and these methods become standardized. Expanding beyond 16S amplification methods using either probes or specific PCR amplicons, larger multiplex tNGS panels will become compelling by allowing for selective amplification and detection of a broad range of pathogens simultaneously without compromising sensitivity and specificity.

As WGS continues to be used, a better understanding of the correlations between AMR detection and phenotypic AST predictions has been gained. However, there is still significant investigation needed to provide a foundation for an accurate alternative for phenotypic AST profiles that are heavily relied on clinically. WGS for *M tuberculosis* complex already shows promise in this area and will likely become standard in the near future. Thus, as simplex continues to be introduced to now highly multiplex PCR AMR panels into the diagnostic arena, one may picture a future where genotypic predictions are introduced without the reliance on phenotype for therapeutic management purposes based on WGS.

For mNGS, more standardization and advancement of methods will be seen for various sample types, including how to interpret and quantify pathogens in samples with complex microbiota (ie, respiratory, urine). Furthermore, one is likely to see these tests converted into precision medicine diagnostics that integrate pathogen, microbiome, and host transcriptome studies to better define the disease state. To support appropriate use and interpretation, there is a need for precision medicine teams that can ensure appropriate test utilization and interpret results. These teams will consist of representatives from clinical microbiology, computational biology, infectious diseases, and other clinician groups, that can contextualize findings in individual patients similar to tumor boards.

There is great momentum for the introduction of NGS applications in clinical microbiology laboratories. Over the next 5 to 10 years, although it is unlikely to see NGS completely supplant traditional identification and AST methods, a wealth of applications must be acquired that is continually improved over time, providing enhanced diagnostic capabilities for patients.

REFERENCES

1. Gu W, Miller S, Chiu CY. Clinical metagenomic next-generation sequencing for pathogen detection. Annu Rev Pathol 2019;14:319–38.

2. Weterings V, Zhou K, Rossen JW, et al. An outbreak of colistin-resistant Klebsiella pneumoniae carbapenemase-producing Klebsiella pneumoniae in The Netherlands (July to December 2013), with inter-institutional spread. Eur J Clin Microbiol Infect Dis 2015;34(8):1647–55.

3. Zhou K, Lokate M, Deurenberg RH, et al. Characterization of a CTX-M-15 producing Klebsiella pneumoniae outbreak strain assigned to a novel sequence type (1427). Front Microbiol 2015;6:1250.

4. Tamma PD, Fan Y, Bergman Y, et al. Applying rapid whole-genome sequencing to predict phenotypic antimicrobial susceptibility testing results among carbapenem-resistant Klebsiella pneumoniae clinical isolates. Antimicrob Agents Chemother 2019;63(1) [pii:e01923-18].

5. Wilson MR, Naccache SN, Samayoa E, et al. Actionable diagnosis of neuroleptospirosis by next-generation sequencing. N Engl J Med 2014;370(25): 2408–17.

6. Brown AC, Bryant JM, Einer-Jensen K, et al. Rapid whole-genome sequencing of Mycobacterium tuberculosis isolates directly from clinical samples. J Clin Microbiol 2015;53(7):2230–7.

7. Votintseva AA, Bradley P, Pankhurst L, et al. Same-day diagnostic and surveillance data for tuberculosis via whole-genome sequencing of direct respiratory samples. J Clin Microbiol 2017;55(5):1285–98.

8. Nimmo C, Doyle R, Burgess C, et al. Rapid identification of a Mycobacterium tuberculosis full genetic drug resistance profile through whole genome sequencing directly from sputum. Int J Infect Dis 2017;62:44–6.

9. Sammons JS, Graf EH, Townsend S, et al. Outbreak of adenovirus in a neonatal intensive care unit: critical importance of equipment cleaning during inpatient ophthalmologic examinations. Ophthalmology 2019;126(1):137–43.

10. Grad YH, Lipsitch M, Feldgarden M, et al. Genomic epidemiology of the Escherichia coli O104:H4 outbreaks in Europe, 2011. Proc Natl Acad Sci U S A 2012;109(8):3065–70.

11. Jackson BR, Tarr C, Strain E, et al. Implementation of nationwide real-time whole-genome sequencing to enhance listeriosis outbreak detection and investigation. Clin Infect Dis 2016;63(3):380–6.

12. Prevention CfDCa. Antibiotic/antimicrobial resistance 2019. 2019. Available at: https://www.cdc.gov/drugresistance/solutions-initiative/index.html. Accessed January 3, 2019.

13. Eyre DW, Cule ML, Wilson DJ, et al. Diverse sources of C. difficile infection identified on whole-genome sequencing. N Engl J Med 2013;369(13):1195–205.

14. Etienne KA, Roe CC, Smith RM, et al. Whole-genome sequencing to determine origin of multinational outbreak of Sarocladium kiliense bloodstream infections. Emerg Infect Dis 2016;22(3):476–81.

15. Leopold SR, Goering RV, Witten A, et al. Bacterial whole-genome sequencing revisited: portable, scalable, and standardized analysis for typing and detection of virulence and antibiotic resistance genes. J Clin Microbiol 2014;52(7):2365–70.

16. Safi H, Lingaraju S, Amin A, et al. Evolution of high-level ethambutol-resistant tuberculosis through interacting mutations in decaprenylphosphoryl-β-D-arabinose biosynthetic and utilization pathway genes. Nat Genet 2013;45(10):1190–7.

17. Power RA, Davaniah S, Derache A, et al. Genome-wide association study of HIV whole genome sequences validated using drug resistance. PLoS One 2016;11(9):e0163746.

18. Tzou PL, Ariyaratne P, Varghese V, et al. Comparison of an in vitro diagnostic next-generation sequencing assay with Sanger sequencing for HIV-1 genotypic resistance testing. J Clin Microbiol 2018;56(6) [pii:e00105-18].

19. Tyson GH, McDermott PF, Li C, et al. WGS accurately predicts antimicrobial resistance in Escherichia coli. J Antimicrob Chemother 2015;70(10):2763–9.

20. Martin J, Phan HTT, Findlay J, et al. Covert dissemination of carbapenemase-producing Klebsiella pneumoniae (KPC) in a successfully controlled outbreak: long- and short-read whole-genome sequencing demonstrate multiple genetic modes of transmission. J Antimicrob Chemother 2017;72(11):3025–34.

21. Nguyen M, Brettin T, Long SW, et al. Developing an in silico minimum inhibitory concentration panel test for Klebsiella pneumoniae. Sci Rep 2018;8(1):421.

22. Jaillard M, van Belkum A, Cady KC, et al. Correlation between phenotypic antibiotic susceptibility and the resistome in Pseudomonas aeruginosa. Int J Antimicrob Agents 2017;50(2):210–8.

23. Mason A, Foster D, Bradley P, et al. Accuracy of different bioinformatics methods in detecting antibiotic resistance and virulence factors from Staphylococcus aureus whole-genome sequences. J Clin Microbiol 2018;56(9) [pii:e01815-17].

24. Eyre DW, De Silva D, Cole K, et al. WGS to predict antibiotic MICs for Neisseria gonorrhoeae. J Antimicrob Chemother 2017;72(7):1937–47.

25. Nguyen M, Long SW, McDermott PF, et al. Using machine learning to predict antimicrobial MICs and associated genomic features for nontyphoidal Salmonella. J Clin Microbiol 2019;57(2) [pii:e01260-18].

26. Quan TP, Bawa Z, Foster D, et al. Evaluation of whole-genome sequencing for mycobacterial species identification and drug susceptibility testing in a clinical setting: a large-scale prospective assessment of performance against line probe assays and phenotyping. J Clin Microbiol 2018;56(2) [pii:e01480-17].

27. Walker TM, Kohl TA, Omar SV, et al. Whole-genome sequencing for prediction of Mycobacterium tuberculosis drug susceptibility and resistance: a retrospective cohort study. Lancet Infect Dis 2015;15(10):1193–202.

28. Bradley P, Gordon NC, Walker TM, et al. Rapid antibiotic-resistance predictions from genome sequence data for Staphylococcus aureus and Mycobacterium tuberculosis. Nat Commun 2015;6:10063.

29. Ellington MJ, Ekelund O, Aarestrup FM, et al. The role of whole genome sequencing in antimicrobial susceptibility testing of bacteria: report from the EU-CAST Subcommittee. Clin Microbiol Infect 2017;23(1):2–22.

30. Deurenberg RH, Bathoorn E, Chlebowicz MA, et al. Application of next generation sequencing in clinical microbiology and infection prevention. J Biotechnol 2017;243:16–24.

31. Rhoads DD. Lowering the barriers to routine whole-genome sequencing of bacteria in the clinical microbiology laboratory. J Clin Microbiol 2018;56(9) [pii: e00813-18].

32. Kos VN, Deraspe M, McLaughlin RE, et al. The resistome of Pseudomonas aeruginosa in relationship to phenotypic susceptibility. Antimicrob Agents Chemother 2015;59(1):427–36.

33. Lemon JK, Khil PP, Frank KM, et al. Rapid nanopore sequencing of plasmids and resistance gene detection in clinical isolates. J Clin Microbiol 2017;55(12): 3530–43.

34. Gordon NC, Price JR, Cole K, et al. Prediction of Staphylococcus aureus antimicrobial resistance by whole-genome sequencing. J Clin Microbiol 2014;52(4): 1182–91.

35. Salipante SJ, Hoogestraat DR, Abbott AN, et al. Coinfection of Fusobacterium nucleatum and Actinomyces israelii in mastoiditis diagnosed by next-generation DNA sequencing. J Clin Microbiol 2014;52(5):1789–92.

36. Gu W, Crawford ED, O'Donovan BD, et al. Depletion of abundant sequences by hybridization (DASH): using Cas9 to remove unwanted high-abundance species in sequencing libraries and molecular counting applications. Genome Biol 2016; 17:41.

37. Schlaberg R, Chiu CY, Miller S, et al. Validation of metagenomic next-generation sequencing tests for universal pathogen detection. Arch Pathol Lab Med 2017; 141(6):776–86.

38. Salipante SJ, Sengupta DJ, Cummings LA, et al. Whole genome sequencing indicates Corynebacterium jeikeium comprises 4 separate genomospecies and identifies a dominant genomospecies among clinical isolates. Int J Med Microbiol 2014;304(8):1001–10.

39. Davidson RM, Epperson LE. Microbiome sequencing methods for studying human diseases. Methods Mol Biol 2018;1706:77–90.
40. Sabat AJ, van Zanten E, Akkerboom V, et al. Targeted next-generation sequencing of the 16S-23S rRNA region for culture-independent bacterial identification—increased discrimination of closely related species. Sci Rep 2017;7(1): 3434.
41. Briese T, Kapoor A, Mishra N, et al. Virome capture sequencing enables sensitive viral diagnosis and comprehensive virome analysis. MBio 2015;6(5). e01491-15.
42. Allicock OM, Guo C, Uhlemann AC, et al. BacCapSeq: a platform for diagnosis and characterization of bacterial infections. MBio 2018;9(5) [pii:e02007-18].
43. Williams SH, Cordey S, Bhuva N, et al. Investigation of the plasma virome from cases of unexplained febrile illness in Tanzania from 2013 to 2014: a comparative analysis between unbiased and VirCapSeq-VERT high-throughput sequencing approaches. mSphere 2018;3(4) [pii:e00311-18].
44. Sahoo MK, Lefterova MI, Yamamoto F, et al. Detection of cytomegalovirus drug resistance mutations by next-generation sequencing. J Clin Microbiol 2013; 51(11):3700–10.
45. Blauwkamp TA, Thair S, Rosen MJ, et al. Analytical and clinical validation of a microbial cell-free DNA sequencing test for infectious disease. Nat Microbiol 2019; 4(4):663–74.
46. Simner PJ, Miller HB, Breitwieser FP, et al. Development and optimization of metagenomic next-generation sequencing methods for cerebrospinal fluid diagnostics. J Clin Microbiol 2018;56(9) [pii:e00472-18].
47. Salzberg SL, Breitwieser FP, Kumar A, et al. Next-generation sequencing in neuropathologic diagnosis of infections of the nervous system. Neurol Neuroimmunol Neuroinflamm 2016;3(4):e251.
48. Wilson MR, O'Donovan BD, Gelfand JM, et al. Chronic meningitis investigated via metagenomic next-generation sequencing. JAMA Neurol 2018;75(8):947–55.
49. Pendleton KM, Erb-Downward JR, Bao Y, et al. Rapid pathogen identification in bacterial pneumonia using real-time metagenomics. Am J Respir Crit Care Med 2017;196(12):1610–2.
50. Zhou Y, Wylie KM, El Feghaly RE, et al. Metagenomic approach for identification of the pathogens associated with diarrhea in stool specimens. J Clin Microbiol 2016;54(2):368–75.
51. Ivy MI, Thoendel MJ, Jeraldo PR, et al. Direct detection and identification of prosthetic joint infection pathogens in synovial fluid by metagenomic shotgun sequencing. J Clin Microbiol 2018;56(9) [pii:e00402-18].
52. Thoendel MJ, Jeraldo PR, Greenwood-Quaintance KE, et al. Identification of prosthetic joint infection pathogens using a shotgun metagenomics approach. Clin Infect Dis 2018;67(9):1333–8.
53. Burnham P, Dadhania D, Heyang M, et al. Urinary cell-free DNA is a versatile analyte for monitoring infections of the urinary tract. Nat Commun 2018;9(1):2412.
54. Li Z, Breitwieser FP, Lu J, et al. Identifying corneal infections in formalin-fixed specimens using next generation sequencing. Invest Ophthalmol Vis Sci 2018; 59(1):280–8.
55. Miao Q, Ma Y, Wang Q, et al. Microbiological diagnostic performance of metagenomic next-generation sequencing when applied to clinical practice. Clin Infect Dis 2018;67(suppl_2):S231–40.
56. Hoffmann B, Tappe D, Hoper D, et al. A variegated squirrel bornavirus associated with fatal human encephalitis. N Engl J Med 2015;373(2):154–62.

57. Wilson MR, Suan D, Duggins A, et al. A novel cause of chronic viral meningoencephalitis: Cache Valley virus. Ann Neurol 2017;82(1):105–14.

58. Thoendel M, Jeraldo PR, Greenwood-Quaintance KE, et al. Comparison of microbial DNA enrichment tools for metagenomic whole genome sequencing. J Microbiol Methods 2016;127:141–5.

59. Salter SJ, Cox MJ, Turek EM, et al. Reagent and laboratory contamination can critically impact sequence-based microbiome analyses. BMC Biol 2014;12:87.

60. Abril MK, Barnett AS, Wegermann K, et al. Diagnosis of Capnocytophaga canimorsus sepsis by whole-genome next-generation sequencing. Open Forum Infect Dis 2016;3(3):ofw144.

61. Greninger AL. The challenge of diagnostic metagenomics. Expert Rev Mol Diagn 2018;18(7):605–15.

62. Swaminathan S, Schlaberg R, Lewis J, et al. Fatal Zika virus infection with secondary nonsexual transmission. N Engl J Med 2016;375(19):1907–9.

63. Yan Q, Wi YM, Thoendel MJ, et al. Evaluation of the CosmosID bioinformatics platform for prosthetic joint-associated sonicate fluid shotgun metagenomic data analysis. J Clin Microbiol 2019;57(2) [pii:e01182-18].

64. Langelier C, Kalantar KL, Moazed F, et al. Integrating host response and unbiased microbe detection for lower respiratory tract infection diagnosis in critically ill adults. Proc Natl Acad Sci U S A 2018;115(52):E12353–62.

65. Simner PJ, Miller S, Carroll KC. Understanding the promises and hurdles of metagenomic next-generation sequencing as a diagnostic tool for infectious diseases. Clin Infect Dis 2018;66(5):778–88.

66. Luscombe NM, Greenbaum D, Gerstein M. What is bioinformatics? An introduction and overview. Yearb Med Inform 2001;(1):83–99.

67. Roy S, Coldren C, Karunamurthy A, et al. Standards and guidelines for validating next-generation sequencing bioinformatics pipelines: a joint recommendation of the Association for Molecular Pathology and the College of American Pathologists. J Mol Diagn 2018;20(1):4–27.

Distributed Microbiology Testing
Bringing Infectious Disease Diagnostics to Point of Care

David R. Peaper, MD, PhD[a], Thomas Durant, MD[b],
Sheldon Campbell, MD, PhD[a],*

KEYWORDS

- Point-of-care testing • Microbiology • Rapid testing • Distributed microbiology
- CLIA waived

KEY POINTS

- Point-of-care microbiology is transitioning from methods predominantly using antigen detection to more molecular testing.
- More analytes and more advanced methods, with clinical properties similar to laboratory-based tests, will move to point-of-care testing.
- Point-of-care diagnostics will require extensive IT development and new models of care to achieve their full potential to improve health.

CONTEXT: POINT-OF-CARE TESTING, WHAT, WHERE, WHO, AND WHY?

From the perspective of laboratory professionals, central laboratory testing is the norm, and testing performed outside of a dedicated laboratory is an emerging field fraught with risk and complexity. However, physicians were testing patient specimens near the patient long before laboratories existed[1] (**Fig. 1**). A laboratory is

[A] facility for the biological, microbiological, serologic, chemical, immunohematological, hematological, biophysical, cytologic, pathologic, or other examination of materials derived from the human body for the purpose of providing information for the diagnosis, prevention, or treatment of any disease or impairment of, or the assessment of the health of, human beings. These examinations also include procedures to determine, measure, or otherwise describe the presence or absence of various substances or organisms in the body. Facilities only collecting or

Disclosure: The authors have nothing to disclose.
[a] Department of Laboratory Medicine, Yale School of Medicine, Pathology and Laboratory Medicine, VA Connecticut Health Care, New Haven, CT 06504, USA; [b] Department of Laboratory Medicine, Yale School of Medicine, New Haven, CT 06504, USA
* Corresponding author.
E-mail address: Sheldon.campbell@yale.edu

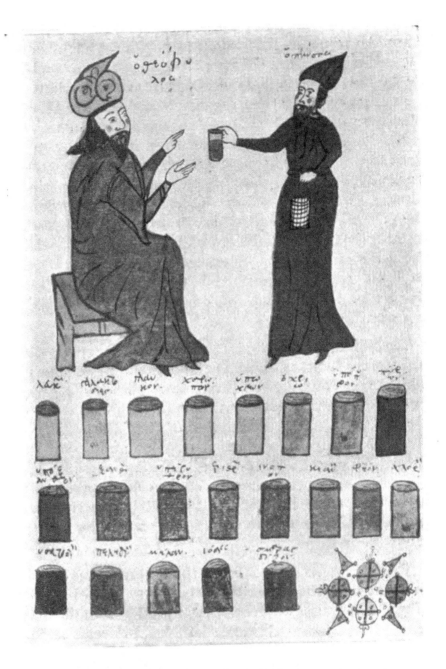

A GREEK PHYSICIAN EXAMINING THE URINE
AND
A DIAGRAM SHOWING THE VARIOUS
COLOURS OF MORBID URINE

Box 1
Some definitions of POCT

College of American Pathologists[29]

Point-of-Care testing (POCT) is defined as tests designed to be used at or near the site where the patient is located, that do not require permanent dedicated space, and that are performed outside the physical facilities of the clinical laboratories. Examples include kits and instruments that are hand carried or otherwise transported to the vicinity of the patient for immediate testing at the site (eg, capillary blood glucose) or analytical instruments that are temporarily brought to a patient care location (eg, operating room, intensive care unit). POCT does NOT include limited service satellite laboratories with fixed dedicated testing space; these are covered under the Limited Service Laboratory Checklist.

A Major Laboratory Medicine Textbook[30]

Point-of-care testing (POCT) is laboratory testing that is, performed outside the central or core laboratory and generally at the site of clinical care or close to the patient. In most settings, POCT is performed by clinical staff rather than laboratorians. Some POCT is also performed by the patient at home.

Wikipedia[31]

Point-of-care testing (POCT), or bedside testing is defined as medical diagnostic testing at or near the point of care—that is, at the time and place of patient care.

---

preparing specimens (or both) or only serving as a mailing service and not performing testing are not considered laboratories.[2]

Point-of-care testing (POCT) is even more difficult to define. The simplest definition is testing performed near or at the patient—the point of care—but, how near is near? Neither the sensitivity nor the specificity of any definition approaches 100%. Some definitions of POCT, used by different sources for different purposes, are found in **Box 1**. Interestingly, the Code of Federal Regulations dealing with clinical laboratory requirements mentions point of care only in passing under Postanalytical Systems: Test Reporting.[2] For the purposes of describing the future of POCT for infectious diseases, we specifically exclude rapid and/or simple tests performed in dedicated laboratory space by dedicated laboratory workers, although this type of testing is directly competitive with POCT and in many cases limits the scope for POCT *sensu stricto*.

In US practice, most POCT performed is Clinical Laboratory Improvement Amendments of 1988 (CLIA) waived. Entities that provide laboratory testing for health assessment or the diagnosis, prevention, or treatment of disease are regulated under CLIA. Waived tests include test systems cleared by the US Food and Drug Administration for home use and those tests approved for waiver under the CLIA criteria.[3] The number of analytes available in CLIA-waived form has increased from 8 in 1992 when the final CLIA rules were approved[4]; as of November of 2018, there were 132 CLIA-waived analytes available.[5] With this explosion of capabilities, one might expect an explosion of applications, with POCT being used to streamline care in many clinical settings. This has not, however, occurred; most laboratory testing is still performed in centralized,

◄─────────────────────────────────────

Fig. 1. A woodcut depicting a Greek physician performing uroscopy, accompanied by a diagram showing the colors of urine in different disease states. (*From* Wellcome HS. The evolution of urine analysis; an historical sketch of the clinical examination of urine. London: Burroughs Wellcome; 1911.)

dedicated laboratories by trained laboratory professionals and then reported back to providers.

What constrains the application of POCT technologies? **Box 2** describes some of the factors we believe set limits on the dissemination of POCT into wider use. The first law describes the human factor; except for medical laboratory professionals, health care workers are untrained in good laboratory practices. Testing systems need to be extraordinarily simple, robust, and reliable for nonlaboratory workers to use them efficiently, and even so, hands-on laboratory testing must be integrated into often busy workflows. The second law describes the placement of POCT within the complex system of health care and the patient encounter; a single laboratory test is only one of many parameters contributing to diagnostic and management decisions, and often is insufficient in itself to drive diagnostic and therapeutic decisions. If a clinical decision requires other laboratory tests or imaging studies that will not be available before a laboratory-generated result is available, a rapid POCT result will have no clinical impact. These factors constrain the dissemination of POCT technologies into routine use.

The range of settings in which POCT is or may be performed is vast, encompassing conventional inpatient, emergency room, and outpatient health care encounters; telemedicinal settings; pharmacies and related outreach community settings; and finally the home. Some of the properties of POCT in these different settings are summarized in **Table 1**. In addition, POCT has the potential for significant impact in low- and middle-income countries, which is covered elsewhere in this volume.

Inpatient care settings typically have on-site laboratories with dedicated testing personnel. Any test that can be performed at POCT can be performed in a laboratory, so any speed advantage of a POCT test is at most the time for transport of the specimen to the laboratory. Some testing (eg, fingerstick glucose) can be performed on capillary blood, which can be obtained more readily than venous blood, and glucose determinations may be useful many times a day. This is unlikely to apply to microbiological testing, however. Currently, few if any microbiology tests are routinely performed at POC for inpatients.

In the emergency department microbiological POCT has more current impact. Emergency department throughput is extremely important for many hospitals; delays in the emergency department can compromise care, are costly, and can harm a

---

Box 2
Campbell's laws of POCT, and corollaries

The Laws

1. Almost nobody goes into medicine or nursing to do diagnostic testing.

2. No POCT, however simple, is easier than filling in one more box on a laboratory order.

The Inpatient Corollary

An inpatient POC test is useful only if:
   The time for transport to the laboratory for THAT SINGLE ANALYTE significantly and negatively impacts care, OR
   The test is performed on an easily obtained sample (eg, fingerstick blood) MORE FREQUENTLY than routine blood draws are obtained.

The Outpatient Corollary

An outpatient POC test is useful only if:
   The test result is available during the patient visit AND a decision can be made or action taken on the basis of it without waiting for other laboratory results, OR
   If you can make money doing it.

Table 1
Microbiological POC in various environments

Care Setting	Clinical Environment	Types of Infections and Problems Seen	Turnaround Time for Impact	Other
Inpatient	Clinical laboratory on-site; often clinically complex patients.	Sepsis; HAI.	Transport time to laboratory has to be long enough to make it worth doing the test at the POC.	Wide range of potential pathogens in many cases.
Emergency	Clinical laboratory on-site	Acute infectious syndromes; some screening.	Test turnaround time strongly impacts throughput.	Tests that can speed discharge strongly favored.
Urgent care	No dedicated laboratory; test availability impacts scope of care available. Space and personnel limited. Volume of testing must justify capital expenses.	Acute infectious syndromes.	Test turnaround time strongly impacts throughput.	Availability of some tests may allow expansion of scope of care available on-site.
Ambulatory	POL on site, or only CLIA-waived tests. Space and personnel limited. Volume of testing must justify capital expenses.	Common health maintenance, screening, and acute ambulatory illnesses.	Test results must be available during the encounter to streamline care.	
Telemedicine	Laboratory may or may not be on-site, depending on the telemedicine model.	Common health maintenance, screening, and acute ambulatory illnesses.	Depends on care model.	Evolving models for telemedicine. In some cases will be linked to other services—pharmacy, imaging. Extent of laboratory tests available at POC may impact scope of care.
Outreach	Specific programs, targeting particular diseases or vulnerable populations. No on-site laboratory; limited, often temporary space.	STI; HIV, HCV.	Rapid—30 min or less for success.	
Home	Patient centered; clinical and interpretive support limited.	STI; acute infectious syndromes; chronic disease screening.	Somewhat flexible; some mail-in testing has been successful.	An evolving area; will expert systems increase the possibilities for home testing?

Abbreviations: HAI, healthcare-associated infection; HCV, hepatitis C virus; HIV, human immunodeficiency virus; POC, point-of-care; POL, physician's office laboratory; STI, sexually transmitted infection.

hospital's reputation.[6] For some diagnoses—for example, uncomplicated influenza, group A streptococcal pharyngitis—extensive laboratory or imaging studies are unnecessary, and the transport of samples to the laboratory may take a significant amount of time, especially in larger facilities. POC flu and group A streptococcus (GAS) testing are frequently performed at the POC in emergency department settings.

In urgent care there is rarely an on-site laboratory. POCT can assist urgent care providers in assessing and managing common infectious syndromes; increasing the analytes available in simple POCT formats may allow urgent care facilities to effectively manage more types of patients.

In the ambulatory care setting, larger practices may have physician's office laboratories with broad capabilities, in dedicated space with dedicated laboratory staff. In less well-equipped settings the limited menu of tests available in CLIA-waived formats limits the application of POCT to:

- Simple syndromes with limited differentials (influenza, pharyngitis, sexually transmitted infection)
- Screening for common conditions (diabetes, hyperlipidemia syndromes, human immunodeficiency virus, hepatitis C virus).
- Management of common therapeutic situations that require frequent monitoring (anticoagulation, diabetes).
- Ancillary testing to assist in rapid assessment of common syndromes (urinalysis)

Although there remain significant gaps in the menu of CLIA-waived tests, a waived complete blood count is now available.[7] The addition of a white blood cell count adds an additional tool to assessment of ambulatory care infectious syndromes[8]; in combination with waived multipathogen respiratory panels, the possibility of ambulatory care triage and management of acute pneumonia is promising. This, however, points out another limiting factor in ambulatory POCT; even CLIA-waived complete blood count and molecular platforms are relatively large instruments with some operating complexity; the investment of space and personnel in this type of equipment needs economic justification and may approach the overhead of a small physician's office laboratory. A proliferation of simple platforms creates its own complexity.

POCT has been used in targeted outreach programs.[9] By their nature, outreach programs, whether aimed at specific diseases (such as human immunodeficiency virus) or at vulnerable populations, benefit from rapid, simple diagnostic systems that can give answers during the encounter, facilitating referrals to care and limiting the need for difficult follow-up processes.

Home testing currently is limited to a small number of simple analytes. The impact of home testing is not well-documented. It is possible that current interest in patient-centered models of care, in combination with connectivity, expert systems, and telemedical interventions, will expand the role of home testing.[10,11]

As point-of-care diagnostics advance, they may change the care delivered in different settings. Similarly, as models of care change, the value of POCT may change with them. These reciprocal impacts are examined in Point-of-care testing in the near future: Strengths, weaknesses, opportunities, and threats.

POINT-OF-CARE TESTING IN THE NEAR FUTURE: STRENGTHS, WEAKNESSES, OPPORTUNITIES, AND THREATS

There is much to love, in theory, about POCT for infectious disease diagnostics, including the provision of an immediate, definitive answer to an acute patient problem (as mentioned, in theory).[12] POC testing for GAS has been a mainstay of clinical practice for decades, and the concept of POC testing in primary care, the emergency room, and urgent care centers is familiar and well-established.[13] Additionally, there have been modeling studies demonstrating the cost effectiveness of the theoretic implementation of different POC assays in different clinical settings beyond standard Ag/Ab assays (**Table 2**).[14]

POC assays for microbiology have historically relied on the detection of bacterial or viral antigens through lateral flow immunoassays with direct visualization of results by the individual performing the testing. Variations in assay format also allow for the detection of antibodies to bacteria or viruses. The recognition that rapid assays for influenza had variable and suboptimal performance prompted increased regulatory scrutiny, which resulted in the withdrawal of a number of tests from the market and the development and release of immunoassays with improved performance.[15] However, these systems are more complex than previous rapid assays and may require the use of readers or other hardware. Simultaneously, advances in nucleic acid amplification tests (NAAT) have occurred such that there are several POC NAAT assays available using polymerase chain reaction and non–polymerase chain reaction NAAT for respiratory pathogens and GAS with excellent sensitivity and specificity.[16] In contrast, POC assays for antibodies have not changed much in recent years. Some non–pathogen-specific tests are also used for POC testing for infectious

Table 2
Strength, weakness, opportunity, and threat (SWOT) analysis of POCT

Strengths	Weaknesses
Everything everyone loves about POC	Instrumentation costs
Not a novel concept to physicians and patients; accustomed to GAS and flu Ag tests	Assay/reagent costs
	Specimen type restrictions (eg, eSwab v. conventional swab)
Current state of the art assays (eg, NAAT, more sensitive Ag assays) have improved performance over past	Serum or plasma beyond POC scope
	Limited infectious disease conditions where aspartate aminotransferase is not relevant
Some POC NAAT comparably sensitive to culture and laboratory-based methods	Quality of testing performance by nonlaboratory staff.
Many clinically relevant specimens readily available: urine, mucosal swabs, whole blood	Arbitrary/limited menus limit clinical impact
	Small number of analytes per platform limit scalability

Opportunities	Threats
Continuing advances in testing: NAAT workflow, turnaround time, lab on a chip	Changes in reimbursement models
	Inertia in physician offices
Antimicrobial stewardship gaining increased importance nationally with regulatory bodies	Theranos effect → Disproportionally increased scrutiny of assays/methods and/or disproportionate fear of regulatory oversight for novel tests/methods
Development of biomarkers for antimicrobial stewardship → Negative Predictive Value	
Development of new antivirals to broaden clinical usefulness (eg, RSV)	Turf wars between pharmacies, urgent cares, offices, emergency departments and potential regulation
Implementing replacement tests at specific, off-site clinics (eg, public health/STI clinics)	
Ability to facilitate new models of care	
Microbiology laboratory consolidation may necessitate more local infectious disease testing	

Abbreviations: NAAT, nucleic acid amplification test; RSV, respiratory syncytial virus.

diseases, including macroscopic urinalysis for urinary tract infection and tests for bacterial vaginosis.

In the near term, the tremendous advances in workflow and turnaround time offered by modern NAAT offer the greatest potential to impact infectious disease POC testing. The replacement of less sensitive Ag methods for influenza and GAS with POC NAAT that do not require supplemental culture or testing by centralized laboratories could occur today. However, there are several barriers to the adoption of these assays by office-based medical practices, including reagent cost, instrument cost, uncertainty regarding reimbursement, and a need to transition to new specimen collection devices (eg, traditional swabs vs eSwabs for GAS). Additionally, the combination of an overworked clinical practice and inertia make the adoption of new tests challenging. The change in US Food and Drug Administration regulations governing rapid influenza antigen tests may speed the uptake of more sensitive POC methods,[14] but that is yet to be seen.

Given these constraints, the biggest opportunity for implementation of existing infectious disease POC NAAT in the near term likely lies in offices and practices that are part of an organized system and/or practice group that could better shoulder the burden of implementation and deal with the financial ambiguity associated with reimbursement of new test methods. Such practices include off-site urgent care centers or offices associated with large health systems or chains. Additionally, if a health system will bear the costs of testing (and benefits of reimbursement) regardless of where testing is performed, the rationale for POC testing can be more easily justified. Finally, as these methods become recognized as the standard of care and reimbursement occurs in a straightforward fashion, their adoption could be a source of revenue for medical offices. However, if reimbursement does not keep pace with testing cost or alternative reimbursement models become more widespread, then the adoption of new methods may be significantly impaired. Uncertainty surrounding test reimbursement is perhaps the biggest threat to the adoption of new testing including POCT.

Current test systems have a narrow test menu that limits their application in POC settings. There are few circumstances where POC tests will be able to replace bacterial culture for the full spectrum of pathogens causing disease, and molecular targets for antimicrobial susceptibility currently cover an extremely limited number of drug/bug combinations. However, research is being conducted to identify and commercialize biomarkers of viral or bacterial infection that could have appropriate negative or positive predictive value to base outpatient antibacterial prescribing decisions. This is especially true for respiratory tract infections in the outpatient setting where antimicrobial stewardship is often in competition with patient satisfaction, including demands for antibiotics. The development of a test to provide reinforcement for antimicrobial stewardship–informed prescribing could affect inappropriate antibacterial usage for upper respiratory tract infections.

Many clinically relevant specimens for syndromes encountered in ambulatory practice are readily obtainable in a POC environment including urine and swabs of mucosal surfaces (eg, pharynx, nasopharynx, and genital). Whole blood, especially finger sticks, is also readily obtainable and commonly used for POC glucose and lead testing. POC tests using whole blood for the detection of antibodies to pathogens are also available. However, serologic testing of whole blood is less widely used than serum, and the extended incubation and/or centrifugation of samples to generate serum or plasma is a challenge for POC engineering.

There is inevitably a chicken-and-egg problem for new laboratory testing, and POC testing is no different: without a market, tests will not be developed, but if there are no tests it is impossible to determine the size of the market. Fortunately, some newer, moderately complex tests can be performed on demand, and studies showing a positive impact on turnaround time for clinical care could be used to justify decentralization to POC environments. The development of a new test for POC use could also lead to novel models for the delivery of care for infections that benefit from urgent treatment or patient populations who may be lost to follow-up. For example, the development of POCT NAAT could significantly streamline the diagnosis and treatment of STIs in emergency departments, urgent care centers, or, most important, public health clinics.

An important factor to consider is that no single POCT platform is capable of performing a full spectrum of relevant infectious disease and noninfectious disease tests for most clinic locations. Among existing analytes, clinical sites may want some combination of GAS, influenza, lead, glucose, hemoglobin A1c, cholesterol, human immunodeficiency virus, and monospot in addition to provider-performed microscopy for wet preps. More acute care locations may also want urine testing for drugs of abuse, lactic acid, blood gases, and other metabolic analytes. Maintaining training and competency on multiple instruments and test systems is a challenge under any circumstance, let alone in direct patient care locations. However, the current state of the market may present an opportunity for a POCT manufacturer to explore integrating infectious disease testing into traditionally noninfectious disease platforms or combining testing methods onto a single instrument with a single workflow for end users. Existing platforms using immunochromatography for the detection of amplified nucleic acid may be such a bridge.[17]

Finally, as microbiology laboratory consolidation continues, there is an opportunity for decentralized microbiology testing to be performed by POCT for appropriate analytes including using POC-like tests in a core laboratory setting. Tests could be implemented locally, thereby providing turnaround time comparable with a location with an on-site microbiology laboratory. However, the greatest opportunities exist in the development and implementation of tests with appropriate positive and negative predictive values to provide clear indications for further testing. Although such tests would be beneficial in almost any clinical setting, their use in a consolidated laboratory system could decrease the amount of packing and shipping of specimens and/or inoculation of culture plates.

INFORMATICS AT THE POINT OF CARE

Lab-on-chip is a general term for describing the miniaturization of currently available laboratory analyzers, which often depend on emerging techniques in microfluidics and microelectronics.[18,19] A current search of the literature and publicly available patents demonstrates an emerging interest in the development of microbiology-related lab-on-chip technology for nucleic acid amplification techniques, lateral flow immunoassays, and others.[20,21] Although the potential applications remain broad, integration and implementation of next-generation POC will surely rely on robust IT solutions and infrastructure, particularly in the setting of infectious disease.

A commonly proposed use case for POCT in microbiology is the usefulness of decentralized testing for public health reporting and disease surveillance.[20] In some instances, POC devices are connected to a data management system that provides integration with traditional laboratory information systems. Currently, disease reporting can be accomplished, even with POC devices, if there is ultimately a connection to a central laboratory information system. However, even in some regions of developed countries, and particularly low- to middle-income countries, POC devices may operate independent of a central laboratory information system, and the usefulness of connectivity with disease surveillance networks becomes apparent.

Although the concept of a decentralized disease surveillance network is undoubtedly appealing, there are special considerations for the design of a decentralized framework, which may benefit from advanced planning. In emerging industry or trending technologies, the pursuit of novel devices or frameworks can quickly lead to unintended product heterogeneity. Similarly, electronic data interchange protocols used to communicate results from POC devices could rapidly devolve into a heterogeneous mixture, precluding facile integration of devices with disease surveillance networks. Similar to the efforts described in current connectivity standards for POC devices published by the Clinical and Laboratory Standards Institute, universal acceptance among vendors should be discussed and promoted early in the development cycle, and in future regulatory and consensus standards, to ensure interoperability between devices and reporting agencies, particularly at an international level.[22]

In 2014, the Clinical and Laboratory Standards Institute published guidelines on IT security and digital transfer of information for in vitro diagnostic devices.[23] For POC devices, which are operating on disease surveillance networks or may require complex postanalytic processing such as artificial intelligence or machine learning, cloud connectivity may be necessary. Because POC devices are often deployed in resource-limited regions, physically secure networks (eg, network cable) are less likely to be available, and broadcast networks (eg, wireless or cellular) or public network communication (eg, the Internet) will be used out of necessity. Accordingly, it should be emphasized to vendors to comply with currently regarded best practices for digital communication over open networks, which may include the implementation of encryption protocols and cryptographic-based messaging.

Computer vision is a subset of artificial intelligence and machine learning that can provide basic classification of digital images when provided a defined scope of potential objects it may encounter, thereby providing the potential for smartphone-based digital microscopy or interpretation of simple, nonautomated tests. For providers practicing in remote locations, computer vision technology is an option for providing automated interpretation of parasites that may be encountered in peripheral blood smears or stool ova and parasite examinations.

Next-generation POC devices, which rely on complex analytics, such as computer vision, will likely require cloud connectivity to optimize processing time, in which case similar concerns about security and data transfer would also apply here.[24]

Last, implementing complex software to support next-generation POC devices in microbiology requires careful consideration of novel validation processes for these complex assays. For any device that may use artificial intelligence, the future of regulatory oversight and best practices for clinical validation remain open questions. In addition, with the potential of increasing complexity of data types (eg, sequencing data), previously published connectivity standards for POC devices may need to be adjusted to accommodate next-generation devices and to ensure universal connectivity.[21]

THE FAR FUTURE: THERANOS, BUT NOT SO STUPID

Managing patients with infectious disease frequently requires laboratory testing beyond pathogen detection to assess clinical severity, exclude other diagnoses, and manage metabolic and systemic complications. It also may require imaging procedures.

Although Theranos' testing model[25] was technologically immature and clinically puerile, the basic concept of moving laboratory testing closer to the site of patient care makes operational sense if it can be done economically and safely. Particularly for routine outpatient medical problems, providing a core menu of routine chemistries, hematology, and microbiological testing at the site of care—probably an emerging care environment that incorporates telemedicine, pharmacy, and possibly imaging as well—will make care more efficient by eliminating the need for follow-up contacts as diagnostic information rolls in, and more effective by completing the assessment, diagnostic testing, and therapeutic phases of care within a single encounter, providing rapid treatment and, probably more important, fewer opportunities for loss to follow-up. Improved diagnostic approaches and biomarkers of infection, as discussed in other articles of this monograph, will contribute, and be incorporated into point-of-care approaches.[26]

The role of clinical laboratories will necessarily evolve as well. Cutting-edge diagnostic technologies will likely always require dedicated laboratories and laboratorians, and the economies of scale for dedicated laboratories will remain compelling for nonurgent analyses and inpatient care. However, an increasingly complex and distributed ambulatory care diagnostic presence will create new opportunities for oversight, training, and quality management for laboratory professionals.

This vision will require technological advances, advanced information technology, and connectivity, and fundamental changes in the model of care.[10,11,27] Rapidly available laboratory testing will have little impact on care if other bottlenecks: availability of imaging, reimbursement, or therapeutics, throttle care pathways. Like all such systems it will evolve through time, planning, and iteration, and will have to evolve as technology, the social matrix, and the microbes themselves evolve.[28] But, modern diagnostics are essential to our current standard of care and moving such diagnostics to POC will be essential to the distributed, patient-centered care model of the mid twenty-first century.

REFERENCES

1. Wellcome HS., 1853-1936The evolution of urine analysis; an historical sketch of the clinical examination of urine. London: Burroughs Wellcome; 1911.

2. Code of federal regulations, 42 CFR Part 943, 'laboratory requirements'. Available at: https://www.ecfr.gov/cgi-bin/text-idx?SID=1248e3189da5e5f936e55315402bc38b&node=pt42.5.493&rgn=div5#se42.5.493_11290. Accessed October 24, 2018.

3. CDC. Clinical Laboratory Improvement Amendments (CLIA). Available at: https://wwwn.cdc.gov/CLIA/Resources/WaivedTests/default.aspx. Accessed November 23, 2018.

4. CDC, minutes of CLIAC meeting in 11/2014. Available at: https://ftp.cdc.gov/pub/CLIAC_meeting_presentations/pdf/Addenda/cliac1114/5a_CLIAC_Waived_Testing_History.pdf. Accessed November 23, 2018.

5. FDA, CLIA - Clinical laboratory improvement amendments - Currently waived analytes. Available at: https://www.accessdata.fda.gov/scripts/cdrh/cfdocs/cfClia/analyteswaived.cfm. Accessed November 23, 2018.

6. McHugh M, Van Dyke K, McClelland M, et al. Improving patient flow and reducing emergency department crowding: a guide for hospitals. Agency for Healthcare Research and Quality Publication No. 11(12)-0094. 2011. Available at: https://www.ahrq.gov/sites/default/files/publications/files/ptflowguide.pdf. Accessed November 23, 2018.

7. US Food and Drug Administration. FDA clears common blood cell count test that offers faster results for patients and providers. 2017. Available at: https://www.fda.gov/NewsEvents/Newsroom/PressAnnouncements/ucm583997.htm. Accessed December 3, 2018.

8. Ellison RT, Donowitz GR. Acute pneumonia. In: Bennett JE, Dolin R, Blaser MJ, editors. Mandell, Douglas, and Bennett's principles and practices of infectious diseases. 8th edition. Philadelphia: Elsevier Churchill Livingstone; 2015. p. 774–83.

9. Thornton AC, Delpech V, Kall MM, et al. HIV testing in community settings in resource-rich countries: a systematic review of the evidence. HIV Med 2012; 13(7):416–26.

10. Heintzman ND. A digital ecosystem of diabetes data and technology: services, systems, and tools enabled by wearables, sensors, and apps. J Diabetes Sci Technol 2015;10(1):35–41.

11. Milani RV, Lavie CJ. Health care 2020: reengineering health care delivery to combat chronic disease. Am J Med 2015;128(4):337–43.

12. Drancourt M, Michel-Lepage A, Boyer S, et al. The point-of-care laboratory in clinical microbiology. Clin Microbiol Rev 2016;29(3):429–47.

13. Dolen V, Bahk K, Carroll KC, et al. Changing diagnostic paradigms for microbiology: report on an American Academy of Microbiology Colloquium held in Washington, DC, from 17 to 18 October 2016. Washington, DC: American Society for Microbiology; 2017.

14. Vecino-Ortiz AI, Goldenberg SD, Douthwaite ST, et al. Impact of a multiplex PCR point-of-care test for influenza A/B and respiratory syncytial virus on an acute pediatric hospital ward. Diagn Microbiol Infect Dis 2018;91(4):331–5.

15. Green DA, StGeorge K. Rapid antigen tests for influenza: rationale and significance of the FDA reclassification. J Clin Microbiol 2018;56(10) [pii:e00711-18].

16. Basile K, Kok J, Dwyer DE. Point-of-care diagnostics for respiratory viral infections. Expert Rev Mol Diagn 2018;18(1):75–83.

17. Faron ML, Ledeboer NA, Granato P, et al. Detection of group A streptococcus in pharyngeal swab specimens by use of the AmpliVue GAS isothermal helicase-dependent amplification assay. J Clin Microbiol 2015;53(7):2365–7.

18. Jung W, Han J, Choi J-W, et al. Point-of-care testing (POCT) diagnostic systems using microfluidic lab-on-a-chip technologies. Microelectron Eng 2015;132: 46–57.

19. Mauk MG, Song J, Liu C, et al. Simple approaches to minimally-instrumented, microfluidic-based point-of-care nucleic acid amplification tests. Biosensors (Basel) 2018;8(1) [pii:E17].

20. Mousavi MZ, Chen H-Y, Lee K-L, et al. Urinary micro-RNA biomarker detection using capped gold nanoslit SPR in a microfluidic chip. Analyst 2015;140(12): 4097–104.

21. Kozel TR, Burnham-Marusich AR. Point-of-care testing for infectious diseases: past, present, and future. J Clin Microbiol 2017;55(8):2313–20.

22. Clinical and Laboratory Standards Institute. POCT01-A2 point-of-care connectivity; approved standard. 2nd edition. Wayne, PA: Clinical and Laboratory Standards Institute; 2006.

23. Clinical and Laboratory Standards Institute. AUTO11-A2 information technology security of in vitro diagnostic instruments and software systems; approved standard. 2nd edition. Wayne, PA: Clinical and Laboratory Standards Institute; 2014.

24. Madabhushi A, Lee G. Image analysis and machine learning in digital pathology: challenges and opportunities. Med Image Anal 2016;33:170–5.

25. Carreyrou J. Bad blood: secrets and lies in a Silicon Valley startup. New York: Alfred A. Knopf; 2018.
26. Waltz E. After Theranos. Nat Biotechnol 2017;35(1):11–5.
27. Parker ML, Yip PM, DeCherrie LV, et al. There's No place like home: exploring home-based, acute-level healthcare. Clin Chem 2018;64(8):1136–42.
28. Hays JP, Mitsakakis K, Luz S, et al, JPIAMR AMR-RDT Consortium. The successful uptake and sustainability of rapid infectious disease and antimicrobial resistance point-of-care testing requires a complex 'mix-and-match' implementation package. Eur J Clin Microbiol Infect Dis 2019;38(6):1015–22. Accessed February 20, 2019.
29. College of American Pathologists, Commission on Laboratory Accreditation, Laboratory Accreditation Program, "Point of care testing" 2017 checklist edition.
30. McVoy L, Lifshitz MS. Point-of-care testing and physician office laboratories. In: McPherson RA, Pincus MR, editors. Henry's clinical diagnosis and management by laboratory methods. 23rd edition. Elsevier; 2017. p. 66–72.
31. "Point of care testing" in Wikipedia. Available at: https://en.wikipedia.org/wiki/Point-of-care_testing. Accessed October 24, 2018.

Direct-from-Specimen Pathogen Identification
Evolution of Syndromic Panels

Marc Roger Couturier, PhD, D(ABMM)[a],*,
Jennifer Dien Bard, PhD, D(ABMM)[b]

KEYWORDS

- Syndromic panel • Respiratory panel • Sepsis panel • Gastroenteritis panel
- Meningitis panel • Encephalitis panel

KEY POINTS

- Syndromic panels should evolve to include additional pathogen targets.
- Syndromic panels should be flexible in design to better meet the user's needs.
- Syndromic panels should include host response markers to correlate with pathogen detection.
- Syndromic panels should have shorter run times, less complexity, and be placed near the point of care.
- Syndromic panels should be expanded to include more antimicrobial resistance determinants and phenotypic susceptibility results.

INTRODUCTION

Clinical laboratory testing for pathogens associated with a specific syndrome have historically relied on multiple different analytical approaches to maximize broad pathogen detection. This is especially true for organisms for which culture was not a feasible modality, and instead culture-independent methods such as antigen detection, direct staining, or targeted polymerase chain reaction (PCR) were the aggregate conventional methods. Since the late 2000s, commercial manufacturers of in vitro diagnostic products have invested significant resources into the development of

Disclosure Statement: M.R. Couturier receives household income from BioFire diagnostics and is involved in clinical trials activities with Luminex (Verigene). J.D. Bard is a consultant for Bio-Fire Diagnostics and Accelerate Diagnostics and is involved in clinical trials activities with Bio-Fire Diagnostics, Luminex Corporation and DiaSorin Molecular.
[a] ARUP Laboratories, University of Utah, 500 Chipeta Way, Salt Lake City, UT 84108, USA;
[b] Microbiology and Virology Laboratories, Department of Pathology and Laboratory Medicine, Children's Hospital Los Angeles, University of Southern California, 4650 Sunset Boulevard MS#32, Los Angeles, CA 90027, USA
* Corresponding author.
E-mail address: marc.couturier@aruplab.com

multiplex molecular diagnostic assays that are capable of detecting a broad array of pathogens that collectively could cause a single clinical syndrome. This became known as the syndromic panel approach to pathogen testing, and this avenue of test design and development has carried through the recent decade with an ever-growing portfolio of offerings from various in vitro diagnostic manufacturers.

Syndromic testing has carried the field of clinical microbiology to a new frontier of diagnostic capabilities. Although many of the advantages of syndromic testing have been met with equal and opposite disadvantages and challenges, a common opinion is that molecular methodologies for many conventional infections are more accurate, rapid, and convenient than most traditional culture and direct detection techniques previously used by laboratories. But what is next and what should the future of these syndromic panels look like? Where are the gaps and what are the unmet needs? This article describes the current state-of-the-art with regards to commercially available (primary those cleared by the US Food and Drug Administration [FDA]) syndromic panels for respiratory tract infections, gastrointestinal (GI) pathogen detection, blood stream infections, and central nervous system (CNS) infections, while providing a pro-vocative and speculative look into the future of syndromic panel testing for infectious diseases.

RESPIRATORY TRACT SYNDROMIC PANELS

Respiratory tract infection panels were the first example of syndromic testing to become commercially available to clinical laboratories approximately 10 or more years ago on a limited number of platforms that have since increased to include multiple different platforms and panel designs. These assays target upper respiratory tract (URT) pathogens from nasopharyngeal swabs or lower respiratory tract patho-gens from aspirates or bronchial lavages. The lower respiratory tract panels (**Table 1**) have only recently been introduced to clinical care, and therefore they are not discussed in detail owing to the unclear nature of their future needs.

Upper Respiratory Tract Panels

URT syndromic testing was a welcomed replacement for insensitive and cumbersome viral cultures and stains as well as imperfect bacterial serology assays. Although PCR for influenza was available to laboratories previously, syndromic panels expanded the detection capacity to include a broad array of common viral targets and select bacteria not traditionally detected by culture. These assays vary in terms of breadth and scope of targets (**Table 2**). The platform ease of use and complexity is also variable. Extreme ends of the spectrum include the BioFire FilmArray Respiratory EZ panel (Bio-Fire Diagnostics, Salt Lake City, UT, USA), which is Clinical Laboratory Improvement Amendments of 1988 waived and can be performed at near point of care, versus the Luminex NxTAG Respiratory Pathogen Panel (Luminex Corporation, Austin, TX USA), which is high complexity and requires molecular laboratory expertise and workspace.

Future target consideration

Emerging respiratory viruses such as enterovirus D68 and coronavirus family mem-bers have been identified recently in outbreaks affecting multiple countries.[1,2] These emerging and evolving viruses pose the most immediate opportunity for assays to provide more comprehensive detection of respiratory viruses. The FilmArray RP2Plus panel currently includes the Middle East respiratory syndrome coronavirus; however, the clinical performance is not fully understood owing to limited widespread circulation of the virus. This target is suppressed in patients who do not meet clinically compatible presentations. This opens up an interesting future opportunity for flexible testing

Table 1
Syndromic panels currently cleared by the US FDA for detection of lower respiratory tract pathogens associated with pneumonia

	FilmArray	Curetis
	Pneumonia Panel	**Hospitalized Pneumonia Panel**
Shared bacterial targets	Staphylococcus aureus[a]	S aureus
	Streptococcus pneumoniae[a]	S pneumoniae
	Proteus spp.[a]	P spp.
	Klebsiella aerogenes[a]	K aerogenes
	Klebsiella pneumoniae group[a]	K pneumoniae
	Klebsiella oxytoca[a]	K oxytoca
	Serretia marcescens[a]	Serretia marcescens
	Moraxella catarrhalis[a]	M catarrhalis
	Pseudomonas aeruginosa[a]	P aeruginosa
	Acinetobacter calcoaceticus-baumannii complex[a]	Acinetobacter baumannii complex
	Haemophilus influenzae[a]	H influenzae
	Mycoplasma pneumoniae	M pneumoniae
	Chlamydophila pneumoniae	C pneumoniae
	Legionella pneumoniae	L pneumoniae
Unique bacterial targets	Streptococcus pyogenes[a]	Stenotrophomonas maltophila
	Streptococcus agalactiae[a]	Morganella morganii
	Escherichia coli[a]	Klebsiella variicola
		Citrobacter freundii
Resistance determinants		tem
		shv
		ermB
	mecA/C	mecA
	MREJ	mecC
	ctx-M	ctx-M
	imp	imp
	kpc	kpc
	ndm	ndm
	vim	vim
	Oxa-48-like	
		oxa-23
		oxa-24/40
		oxa-48
		oxa-58
		sul1
		gyrA83
		gryA87
Viral or fungal targets	Adenovirus	Pneumocystis jirovecii
	Coronavirus	
	Human metapneumovirus	
	Human rhinovirus/enterovirus	
	Influenza A	
	Influenza B	
	Parainfluenza virus	
	Respiratory syncytial virus	

[a] Bacterial targets are reported semiquantitative.

Table 2
Syndromic panels currently cleared by the US FDA for detection of URT pathogens

Target Organism	FilmArray		Verigene	Luminex			GenMark	
	RP	RP EZ	RP Flex	xTAG RVP	xTAG RVP Fast v2	NxTAG RPP	XT-8 RVP	ePlex RP
Viruses								
Respiratory syncytial virus	•	•			•			
Respiratory syncytial virus A			•	•		•	•	•
Respiratory syncytial virus B			•	•		•	•	•
Influenza A	•	•	•		•	•	•	•
Influenza A matrix				•	•			
H1 subtype	•	•	•	•	•	•	•	•
H3 subtype	•	•	•	•	•	•	•	•
H1-2009 subtype	•	•					•	•
Influenza B	•	•	•	•	•	•	•	•
Parainfluenza virus		•						
Parainfluenza 1	•		•	•	•	•	•	•
Parainfluenza 2	•		•	•		•	•	•
Parainfluenza 3	•		•	•		•	•	•
Parainfluenza 4	•		•					•
Human metapneumovirus	•	•	•	•	•	•	•	•
Adenovirus	•	•	•	•	•	•		•
Adenovirus C							•	

Adenovirus B/E

Human rhinovirus/enterovirus

Human rhinovirus

Coronavirus

Coronavirus HKU1

Coronaovirus NL63

Coronavirus 229E

Coronavirus OC43

MERS coronavirus[a]

Human bocavirus

Bacteria

Mycoplasma pneumoniae

Chlamydia pneumoniae

Bordetella pertussis

Bordetella parapertussis[b]

Bordetella parapertussis/B bronchiseptica

Bordetella holmesii

•, Panel is cleared by the FDA to detect this pathogen.
[a] Available on RP2 PLUS (Not cleared by US FDA).
[b] Available on RP2.

options related to such pathogens. Because the positive predictive value of a test result will be significantly impaired in the absence of circulating virus, emerging respiratory pathogens (eg, Middle East respiratory syndrome coronavirus, enterovirus D68, severe acute respiratory syndrome) could be included in a syndromic panel, but the end-user could have the option of disabling this target in the absence of documented circulation.

Surveillance potential for novel pathogens

An alternative approach could be that certain targets could be tested but not immediately visible. The results could instead be communicated to the manufacturer through a cloud-based surveillance system. In this way, a sporadic false positive could be easily identified, but a community-level cluster of positives could be identified by the manufacturer and an investigation and communication with the end-user laboratories and treating physicians could ensue. Although this may be an Orwellian, intrusive system, a similar voluntary surveillance system already exists for BioFire users and could have value in future epidemiologic outbreak identification.[3] Rather than continuing to chase outbreaks after the fact, earlier crowd sharing of silent surveillance data could serve the entire community while not sounding an alarm on a sporadic false-positive result. This process would require a discussion of who pays for this extra effort and target detection—manufacturers, public health, or end-users.

Simple, rapid, and near point-of-care testing

The future of URT pathogen testing is ultimately coming to near point-of-care with extremely rapid turn around time. Although microbiology laboratories are hesitant to let go of their testing fiefdom, the logical progression of testing and rapid decision making lies in having answers immediately available and actionable. Examples of technologies that bring single or 2-target respiratory pathogen testing to near point of care for influenza have been embraced in many health care settings (despite imperfect performance characteristics) and have allowed for more efficient use of emergency rooms and decreased costs.[4,5] Comprehensive URT panels with even shorter turn around time than current assays could allow for improved management of admissions and patient cohorting, while possibly reducing early empiric (and often unnecessary) antibiotic administration.

GASTROINTESTINAL SYNDROMIC PANELS

GI pathogen detection has historically relied upon multiple classic complementary diagnostics modalities (eg, culture, fecal antigen detection, microscopy, single target PCR) to create a comprehensive pseudopanel of targets. A longstanding challenge with respect to GI pathogen detection includes multiple factors:

1. Limited capacities of the local laboratory and lack of usefulness for reference laboratory testing for acute GI illness
2. Physician ordering lapses stemming from a lack of understanding of test methods and detection capabilities
3. Preanalytical and analytical factors that decrease sensitivity of the available methods (eg, delayed transport or preservation of stool, inexperienced technologists, general unfamiliarity with less frequently encountered pathogens)

Syndromic panels have approached these challenges by compartmentalizing pathogens into a single large panel or multiple modular panels grouped by taxonomic relatedness (eg, bacteria, viruses, protozoa).

Modular Panels

Small modular panels can detect more common bacteria, viruses, or protozoa. These panels for the most part have targeted the highest prevalence or significance organism at the expense of less comprehensive detection of other pathogens. A panel capable of detecting *Salmonella*, *Shigella*, *Campylobacter jejuni/coli*, and Shiga-like toxin genes of Shiga-toxigenic *Escherichia coli* was essentially a replacement for conventional stool culture. However, clinical concerns about failing to detect less frequently encountered pathogens such as *Vibrio*, *Yersinia entrocolitica*, and enterotoxigenic *E coli* drove the creation of expanded bacterial panels which could be considered for specific patient populations or patients who initially test negative for the more common bacterial pathogens (**Table 3**).

Similarly, standalone parasitic panels primarily targeting the most common protozoal pathogens can be viewed as replacements for stool ova and parasite examinations, with only a rare subset of patients requiring a full ova and parasite examination to rule out helminth infections or less common protozoal pathogens (eg, *Cystoisospora*, *Balantidioides*). The most common configuration of testing includes *Giardia*, *Cryptosporidium*, and *Entamoeba histolytica* (see **Table 3**).

Modular panels for enteric viral pathogens have not been widely commercialize to date, with only 1 product from BD (Beckton Dickinson, Franklin Lakes, NJ, USA) having clearance from the FDA (see **Table 3**). This may be understandable from a practical standpoint because conventional testing for GI viruses has not been universally embraced as a standard of care, with the exception of rotavirus antigen detection for neonates and PCR for noroviruses in outbreak settings.[6]

Table 3 Modular panels currently cleared by the US FDA for detection of GI pathogens currently cleared by the US FDA		
Target Organism	**BDMax**	**Prodesse**
Bacterial		
Campylobacter	•	‡
Salmonella	•	‡
Shigella	•	‡
Shiga-like toxin 1 and 2 (STEC)	•	‡
Enterotoxigenic *Escherichia coli*	*	
Vibrio	*	
Yersinia enterocolitica	*	
Plesiomonas shigelloides	*	
Parasitic		
Giardia	+	
Cryptosporidium	+	
Entamoeba histolytica	+	
Viral		
Norovirus	††	
Adenovirus (40/41)	††	
Rotavirus	††	
Astrovirus	††	
Sapovirus	††	

-, enteric bacterial panel; *, extended bacterial panel; +, enteric parasite panel; ††, enteric viral panel; ‡, ProGastro SSCS.

Comprehensive Panel

Several commercial panels are capable of detecting bacteria, viruses, and protozoa in a single assay (**Table 4**). These panels vary by specific target in the case of bacteria and viruses; however, a core set of pathogen targets has been included in most commercial assays. These targets are thought to represent the most common enteric pathogens.

Existing Gaps

Targets of unclear or unestablished significance

To date, GI panels have included definitive pathogens; however, some detect organisms with less definitively established pathogenicity. Such targets include enteroaggregative *E coli*, enteropathogenic *E coli*, and *Plesiomonas shigelloides*. Manufacturers should consider removing or masquing such targets or conducting additional clinical studies to better establish significance in specific test populations before integrating them into the panels.

Table 4
Syndromic, broad panels currently cleared by the US FDA for GI pathogen detection

Target Organism	FilmArray GI Panel	Verigene Enteric Pathogens Test	Luminex GI Pathogens Panel
Bacterial			
Campylobacter	•	•	•
Salmonella	•	•	•
Shigella	•	•	•
Shiga-like toxin 1 and 2	•	•[a]	•
Enterotoxigenic Escherichia coli	•		•
Enteropathogenic E coli	•		
Enteroaggregative E coli	•		
E coli O157	•		•
Vibrio	•	•	
Yersinia enterocolitica	•	•	
Plesiomonas shigelloides	•		
Clostridium difficile	•		•
Viral			
Norovirus GI and GII	•	•	•
Adenovirus 40/41	•		•
Rotavirus	•	•	•
Astrovirus	•		
Sapovirus	•		
Parasitic			
Giardia	•		•
Cryptosporidium	•		•
Cyclospora cayetanensis	•		
Entamoeba histolytica	•		•

•, Panel is cleared by the FDA to detect this pathogen.
[a] Verigene detects and reports each shiga-like toxin gene separately.

Targets with clinical relevance but not universally included

A glaring hole in the design of most commercial assays is the notable exclusion of *Cyclospora cayetanensis*. This pathogen is of significant importance in the Americas and in the recent decade has become a quasiseasonal illness in the United States owing to imported produce serving as a vehicle for multistate and nationwide outbreaks. One study has already demonstrated the value of detecting *C cayetanensis* directly from stool specimens during an outbreak.[7] Despite this prevalence and clinical/epidemiologic significance, the target has been excluded from multiple panels in favor of *E histolytica* (see **Tables 3** and **4**). Although *E histolytica* is a virulent protozoal pathogen, its incidence is very low in developed countries. In this author's laboratory, *Cyclospora* is the most frequently detected protozoal pathogen and *E histolytica* ranks fifth of the 5 protozoa detected by a syndromic panel. Furthermore, some commercial assays are not able to specifically identify *E histolytica* from the nonpathogenic *Entamoeba dispar*. This limitation is essentially the same problem that has plagued ova and parasite examinations for a century. Improving the species-level specificity for *E histolytica* and inclusion of *Cyclospora* in future products is imperative.

Clostridioides difficile testing without clinical indication

Testing for *C difficile* has been an area of clinical diagnosis that has evolved significantly over the past decade. Although the nuances and opinions with regard to this infection are beyond the scope of this work, there are some practical issues that arise as a result of panel tests that include this target. Testing for *C difficile* in children less than 24 months of age has been traditionally discouraged because children in this age group are often asymptomatically colonized.[8] Furthermore, testing for *C difficile* in otherwise healthy adult populations without previous use of antibiotics or hospitalization or hospital exposure has not historically been advocated during primary clinical evaluations.[8] Inclusion of this target can increase the risk for further overdiagnosis of *C difficile*.

Host response targeting

Another future area of consideration for aiding in the interpretation of colonization versus infectious state could include the integration of mucosal inflammatory marker expression, for example, proinflammatory cytokines. Markers of acute inflammation could serve as an adjunct metric to aid in interpreting the detection of potential colonizers like *C difficile* or organisms capable of shedding for week or month after convalescence (eg, *Salmonella* and norovirus). This would be an area still in need of significant research because molecular profiling for inflammatory bowel disease and other similar conditions is not yet a standard of care.

Demographic and region-specific testing

Demographic or region-specific assays (or convenient end-user customization) should be an area of future consideration for manufacturers. Future GI syndromic testing must be customizable to fit the needs of the individual laboratory or region while not overtesting for targets that have low to no prevalence in the region or demographic. For example, although including *Cyclospora* in a syndromic panel may be very relevant for the Americas and tropical/subtropical countries, it may be a completely unnecessary target in other regions (eg, Canada, Northern and Eastern Europe). Although rare infections may be encountered in these regions, it may not be cost effective to test all specimens for this target and in the absence of true infections, the positive predictive value of this target will be poor. Considering demographic-driven testing, a community hospital with primarily uncomplicated patients would have a different pathogen list to consider for clinical care than a large academic medical center that supports a transplant center, human immunodeficiency virus clinic, and travel/tropical medicine clinic.

A flexible end-user design already exists in the Verigene (Luminex Corp., Austin, TX, USA) RP Flex assay.

Detection of antimicrobial resistance

One challenge that is unmet by the current GI syndromic testing is the detection of antimicrobial resistance to primary empiric antibiotics. This is a daunting technical challenge in a specimen such as stool that contains copious genera of commensal microbiota; however, even a few targets for primary resistance could be invaluable to clinical care for some enteric bacterial pathogens. Organisms such as *Shigella*, *Salmonella*, and *Campylobacter* are currently cultured after syndromic testing in efforts to maintain public health outbreak tracking, but also to provide primary antimicrobial susceptibility testing for selected drug classes in cases of severe infection.[9,10] These organisms often are not culturable after primary syndromic testing, so having markers for macrolide, quinolone, and/or tetracycline resistance could be extremely helpful for treating clinicians and epidemiologic reporting.[11] Clearly this is a technically challenging request and one that may be more idealistic than realistic given current technologies, but should nonetheless be a future target goal for testing.

Gastrointestinal Panel Future Needs Summary

Future syndromic testing for GI pathogens should consider

1. Customizable or regional/demographic-driven targets
2. Inclusion of only clinically relevant targets or those with well-established clinical significance
3. Inclusion of inflammatory markers to aid in identifying potential colonizers versus active infections
4. Inclusion of antimicrobial resistance determinants for outbreak associated bacterial pathogens

BLOODSTREAM SYNDROMIC PANELS

Expeditious identification of bloodstream pathogens through the use of molecular syndromic panels has dramatically altered the standard of care in many laboratories. There are currently 6 FDA-cleared multiplexed assays directly from positive blood cultures (**Table 5**)—4 bacterial panels coupled with resistance determinants, 1 fungal panel, and 1 panel that generates minimum inhibitory concentration in lieu of resistance markers. There are currently 2 direct from whole blood panels.

Future Directions and Considerations

Target wish list

Expansion of existing panels to include additional pathogens and more comprehensive resistance determinants is ongoing. The ePlex BCID-GP panel is currently the most comprehensive panel for gram-positive organisms and also includes pan–gram-negative and pan-*Candida* targets as a safeguard for Gram stain interpretation (see **Table 5**). Additional gram-positive organisms that may be considered are *Streptococcus mitis/oralis*, an important bloodstream infection (BSI) agent in patients with underlying hematologic and oncologic diseases, and *Corynebacterium jeikeium*. The inclusion of targets for *Mycobacterium* species, particularly the rapid-growing nontuberculosis *Mycobacterium*, would also be beneficial for certain patient demographics.

A relatively underappreciated pathogen group are anaerobes, accounting for approximately 20% of BSIs.[12] An up and coming gram-negative panel (BCID-GN) targets numerous obligate anaerobes, including *Fusobacterium necrophorum*, *F nucleatum*,

Table 5
Syndromic, broad panels currently cleared by the US FDA for bloodstream pathogen detection

	BioFire	Luminex		GenMark			Accelerate	T2 BioSystem	
Target Organism	FilmArray BCID[a]	Verigene BC-GN[a]	Verigene BC-GP[a]	ePlex BCID-GN[a]	ePlex BCID-GP[a]	ePlex BCID-FP[a]	PhenoTest BC	T2Candida[b]	T2Bacteria[b]
Gram-negative bacteria									
Acinetobacter species		•							
Acinetobacter baumannii	•						•		
Citrobacter species		•					•		
Enterobacteriaceae	•								
Enterobacter species		•							
Enterobacter cloacae complex	•						•		
Escherichia coli	•	•					•		•
Haemophilus infuenzae	•								
Klebsiella species							•		
Klebsiella oxytoca	•	•							
Klebsiella pneumoniae	•	•							•
Neisseria meningitidis	•								
Pan gram-negative					•				
Proteus species	•	•					•		
Pseudomonas aeruginosa	•	•					•		•
Serratia marcescens	•	•					•		
Gram-positive bacteria									
Bacillus cereus group					•				
Bacillus subtilis group					•				
Corynebacterium					•				
Cutibacterium acnes					•				

(continued on next page)

Table 5
(continued)

Target Organism	BioFire	Luminex		GenMark		Accelerate	T2 BioSystem	
	FilmArray BCID[a]	Verigene BC-GN[a]	Verigene BC-GP[a]	ePlex BCID-GP[a]	ePlex BCID-FP[a]	PhenoTest BC	T2Candida[b]	T2Bacteria[b]
Enterococcus species	•			•				
Enterococcus faecium			•	•		•		•
Enterococcus faecalis			•	•		•		
Lactobacillus species				•				
Listeria species			•	•				
Listeria monocytogenes	•			•				
Micrococcus species				•				
Staphylococcus species	•		•	•		•		
Staphylococcus aureus	•		•	•		•		•
Staphylococcus lugdunensis			•	•		•		
Staphylococcus epidermidis			•	•				
S species	•		•	•		•		
Streptococcus agalactiae	•		•	•				
Streptococcus pyogenes	•		•	•				
Streptococcus anginosus			•	•				
Streptococcus pneumoniae	•		•	•				
Fungal								
Candida albicans					•	•	•	
Candida auris					•			
Candida dubliniensis					•			
Candida famata					•			

Candida glabrata

Candida guilliermondii

Candida keyr

Candida krusei

Candida lusitaniae

Candida parapsilosis

Candida tropicalis

Cryptococcus gattii

Cryptococcus neoformans

Fusarium

Pan Candida

Rhodotorula

Antimicrobial susceptibility testing

Genotypic susceptibility

CTX-M

IMI

KPC

NDM

OXA

VIM

mecA

mecC

vanA/B

Phenotypic susceptibility

Minimum inhibitory concentration*

•, Panel is cleared by the FDA to detect this pathogen.
a Testing on positive blood cultures.
b Testing on whole blood.

and *Bacteriodes fragilis*. Likewise, the next generation of the FilmArray BCID (BCID2) will include *B fragilis*. Inclusion of additional obligate anaerobes (eg, *Clostridium* spp.) would further expand the breadth of coverage offered in these syndromic panels.

The inclusion of select agent targets such as *Brucella* spp, *Franciscella* spp., and *Burkholderia pseudomallei* may prevent unnecessary laboratory exposure. This request may be onerous for manufacturers to fulfill owing to restrictions associated with select agent testing. Last, the development of a fungal panel that includes comprehensive list of molds would significantly improve time to identification. The ePlex BCID-FP panel offers detection of *Fusarium* spp. (see **Table 5**), but some additional relevant targets to consider are *Scedosporium apiospermum* and *Lomentospora prolificans*.

Direct from whole blood testing

There is a crucial unmet need to bypass the primary incubation step entirely. Exciting new technologies are currently in development, and an excellent summary of these technologies are provided by Sinha and colleagues.[13] The first innovative step to this holy grail approach is the release of 2 FDA-cleared, whole blood assays (see **Table 5**) that target 5 bacteria and *Candida* species. This is a significant milestone in BSI diagnostics and provides insight for future panels. For starters, whole blood syndromic testing is an adjunct to conventional blood cultures and manufacturers must consider the pediatric population and associated blood volume limitations. A requirement of less than 1 mL of blood in children would be optimal. Second, the targets incorporated must be analogous to the aforementioned direct from positive blood culture panels. Preferably, a compendious list of bacterial, viral, and fungal pathogens should be offered, without compromising the sensitivity of the test. The ability to detect polymicrobial infections despite low pathogen load is paramount for appropriate antimicrobial coverage. Importantly, the breadth of targets and high sensitivity will allow for high confidence in a negative result to potentially decrease antimicrobial use. An overarching goal is to be as target agnostic as possible while maintaining rapidity.

There are a number of caveats to whole blood syndromic testing that needs to be rectified before widespread adoption. First, the increase risk for contamination exists, particularly if extensive manual manipulation is required. Emerging technologies are attempting to alleviate this risk by innovative approaches, including the use of small reaction mixture volumes to reduce the number of contaminating DNA.[14] Second, current BSI syndromic panels pricing is not conducive to testing on all patients with corresponding blood cultures. Manufacturers must be aware of the budgetary limitations instilled on laboratories that may prohibit adoption. The development of a diagnostic algorithm that integrates host response as a predicate of whole blood syndromic testing may be a potential strategy to distinguish low risk patients from septic patients. The SeptiCyte (Immunexpress Inc., Seattle, WA), a recently FDA-cleared quantitative reverse transcriptase PCR based assay, measures levels of biomarkers (CEACAM4, LAMP1, PLA2G7, and PLAC8) to distinguish between sepsis and noninfectious process in adult patients only.[15] A pilot study of 70 pediatric patients also demonstrated promising results.[16] A noteworthy limitation is the required 2.5 mL for testing and future development of host response assays should also be cognizant of blood volume constraints.

Antimicrobial susceptibility needs

Inarguably, the impact of timely susceptibility results is profound because it allows for antimicrobial optimization. New generations of BSI syndromic panels currently in development have expanded the list of resistance targets of epidemiologic and therapeutic importance including, *mecC* and *mcr-1* genes. However, targets to detect extended-spectrum beta-lactamase production remains limited to the bla_{CTX-M} gene and would benefit from additional genes, including bla_{SHV} and bla_{TEM}.

In contrast with genotypic resistance detection offered by the majority of panels, there is a paucity of rapid phenotypic susceptibility platforms. Although both testing modalities have clinical usefulness, only panels that provide simultaneous identification and phenotypic susceptibility results can function as a standalone test. Expansion of the identification capabilities of the existing PhenoTest BC (Accelerate Diagnostics, Tucson, AZ, USA) would be beneficial, because the gram-positive targets are currently limited (see **Table 5**). Manufacturers need to also be cognizant of prioritizing the release of susceptibility testing options for novel antimicrobial agents and to accommodate clinical breakpoints changes.

Finally, the amalgamation of direct whole blood syndromic panel with phenotypic susceptibility testing is an ambitious request that may be realistically fulfilled in the near few years.

CENTRAL NERVOUS SYSTEM SYNDROMIC PANELS

Laboratory diagnostic tests are compulsory to confirm CNS infection. The diagnostic accuracy of conventional microbiological approaches, such as Gram stain and culture, is hampered by low sensitivity and/or slow turnaround time. New and emerging diagnostic approaches to aid in the diagnosis of meningitis and encephalitis may address the limitations of current laboratory practices.

There are currently only 3 FDA-cleared tests for the detection of pathogens directly from cerebrospinal fluid (CSF) specimens (**Table 6**). The first 2 are limited-target,

Table 6
Syndromic, broad panels currently cleared by the US FDA for meningitis/encephalitis pathogen detection

Target Organism	BioFire FilmArray Meningitis/ Encephalitis	DiaSorin Simplexa HSV 1 and 2 Direct	Cepheid Xpert EV
Bacterial			
Escherichia coli K1	•		
Haemophilus influenzae	•		
Listeria monocytogenes	•		
Neisseria meningitidis	•		
Streptococcus agalactiae	•		
Streptococcus pneumoniae	•		
Viral			
Cytomegalovirus	•		
Enterovirus	•		•
Herpes simplex virus-1	•	•	
Herpes simplex virus-2	•	•	
Human herpes virus-6	•		
Human parechovirus	•		
Varicella zoster virus	•		
Yeast			
Crytococcus neoformans/gattii	•		

•, Panel is cleared by the FDA to detect this pathogen.

qualitative tests that detects 1 to 2 viral pathogens. The final FDA-cleared test is the FilmArray Meningitis/Encephalitis panel, offering simultaneous detection of multiple pathogens from CSF samples. Testing is finite, and conventional culture remains of the utmost importance for the recovery of additional pathogens and for susceptibility testing when appropriate. Other key points about current syndromic testing for CNS infections include:

1. Increased pathogen detection compared with conventional laboratory approaches
2. Associated risks of contamination necessitate the need for strict adherence to molecular testing policies
3. Low viral load in CSF for certain viruses (eg, herpes simplex virus) may warrant additional testing from alternate sources (eg, blood)
4. Molecular testing may be suboptimal for certain pathogens (eg, cryptococcal antigen testing continues to be the diagnostic standard)
5. Detection of herpes viruses could represent either latent or active infection. Chromosomal integration is also a possibility in patients positive for human herpes virus-6 (inherited chromosomally integrated human herpes virus-6).
6. Corroboration of findings with clinical picture is paramount to ensure the most appropriate diagnosis and patient management.

Existing Gaps

Syndromic testing for CNS infections remains in its infancy. Continuous innovation and development are fundamental to the diagnostic advancement of CNS infections. A quick fix that current and future manufacturers may consider would be to decrease the required CSF volume to accommodate the copious numbers of tests often ordered.

Acute versus chronic central nervous system infections
It may be valuable to offer customizable panels for acute versus chronic CNS infections. Acute meningitis is often caused by viruses and bacteria included in the FilmArray Meningitis/Encephalitis panel. In contrast, chronic meningitis can result from infection with *Mycobacterium tuberculosis* and fungal pathogens including, *Aspergillus*, *Histoplasma*, *Blastomyces*, and *Coccidiodes*.[17] The inclusion of additional, uncultivable pathogens, may add further value to the panel (eg, *Bartonella* spp. and *Treponema pallidum*). This demographic consideration can be expanded geographically to include pathogens that may be applicable to certain regions.

Shunt infections
An entire niche of CNS infections remains untouched. Cumulative incidence rates of shunt infections range from 10% to 22% per patient with 90% of infections occurring within 30 days of surgery.[18] No commercial molecular tests exist for the diagnosis of shunt infections and microbiology culture remains the primary approach. The microbiological demographic of shunt infections is attributed to skin flora and differ significantly from patients with acute meningitis and encephalitis. As such, the FilmArray Meningitis/Encephalitis panel is not appropriate for patients with indwelling devices and also not approved by the FDA for such testing. Laboratory-developed molecular tests that detect *Staphylococcus aureus* and *Cutibacterium acnes* from shunt specimens have yielded promising data, including increased detection in patients with prior antimicrobial exposure.[19] We envision future assays that target common shunt pathogens including, *S aureus*, *C acnes*, coagulase-negative staphylococci, gram-negative organisms, and *Candida* spp. A foreseen limitation would be the risk of skin flora contamination, which may impede the inclusion of coagulase-negative staphylococci target.

Testing in cases of mosquito exposure

Arbovirus infections are important causes of neuroinvasive diseases associated with endemic transmission or travel-related mosquito exposures. Molecular testing of CSF specimen may be inferior in cases of arbovirus infections because the window for viral detection is mere days from symptom onset compared with the measurement of IgM and IgG antibody responses, which remain elevated for weeks.[20] Thus, diagnosis is made primarily by serology. However, the superiority of serologic testing may be hampered in immunosuppressed patients, stressing the need for enhanced diagnostic tools.

Recent studies revealed promising results for detection of West Nile virus from whole blood and urine.[21,22] A retrospective study of 38 patients with West Nile virus confirmed superiority of molecular detection of West Nile virus in whole blood compared with CSF with a sensitivity of 86.8% and 16.6%, respectively.[21] Yet molecular testing of CSF specimens may still be valuable.[23] Potential syndromic panel for routine detection of arboviruses may integrate molecular testing from whole blood and CSF alongside serologic testing to improve diagnostic yield.

Syndromic testing paired with cytokine profiling

Owing to an active innate immune system in the CNS that rapidly responds to alterations in CNS homeostasis, the levels of biomarkers and cytokines released into the CSF may be diagnostic discriminators. Future syndromic panels may incorporate molecular target detection alongside markers of host responses. Studies on the role of biomarkers in predicting CNS infections and to differentiate bacterial from viral meningitis is ongoing. CSF lactate may be a promising marker to rule out bacterial meningitis with high sensitivity (93%–95%) and specificity (95%–96%),[24] albeit a significant decrease in sensitivity is noted with antibiotic exposure.[24]

A recent proof-of-concept study using the Luminex FlexMPA 3D technology determined that quantification of cytokine levels in the CSF can rule in or out an infectious process. Specifically, high levels of IP-10/CXCL10 were present in CNS infections and MDC/CCL22 levels were significantly higher in nonviral infections. Deciphering between oncologic process and autoimmune encephalitis may also be possible, as indicated by high levels of GRO/CXCL1, IL-7, and IL-8 in gliomas.[25] A potential steward of diagnostic testing would include screening for infectious processes by cytokine profiling followed by subsequent testing with syndromic panel. This method could potentially provide decipher between latent versus active viral infection or cases of chromosomally integrated human herpes virus-6 (iciHHV-6). Again, the integration of this algorithmic approach must maintain STAT testing capabilities to maximize the benefit of expeditious testing currently offered by syndromic panels. Extensive research is required to determine true clinical performance and usefulness of such tests.

Antimicrobial susceptibility

Inclusions of potential resistance markers and/or direct from specimen phenotypic susceptibility may be beneficial for some CNS pathogens including, *Streptococcus pneumoniae, Haemophilus influenzae*, and *E coli* K1. One example is to establish *H influenzae* antimicrobial profile as beta-lactamase positive, beta-lactamase negative ampicillin susceptible, and beta-lactamase positive ampicillin resistant by the detection of such genes as TEM-1, ROB-1, and PBP3.[26] In line with potential assays for shunt infections, inclusion of *mecA* and *mecC* gene for detection of methicillin resistance in *S aureus* is beneficial. An idealistic request is to develop direct from positive CSF specimen phenotypic susceptibility testing. Future development may consider either a standalone identification and susceptibility testing platform or in collaboration with existing identification platforms to consolidate the susceptibility portion.

SUMMARY

There are numerous areas of opportunity to advance the role of syndromic panels in clinical care for respiratory, GI, blood stream infections, and CNS. Based on the primary points of this article, the future of syndromic testing should include:

1. Refining existing targets and inclusion of emerging pathogen targets
2. Expansion of specimen types and volumes required for testing
3. Integration of host response markers
4. Inclusion of additional antimicrobial resistance determinants and phenotypic susceptibility
5. Simple, fast, near point-of-care platforms

REFERENCES

1. Bialek SR, Allen D, Alvarado-Ramy F, et al. First confirmed cases of Middle East respiratory syndrome coronavirus (MERS-CoV) infection in the United States, updated information on the epidemiology of MERS-CoV infection, and guidance for the public, clinicians, and public health authorities - May 2014. MMWR Morb Mortal Wkly Rep 2014;63(19):431–6.
2. Midgley CM, Jackson MA, Selvarangan R, et al. Severe respiratory illness associated with enterovirus D68 - Missouri and Illinois, 2014. MMWR Morb Mortal Wkly Rep 2014;63(36):798–9.
3. Meyers L, Ginocchio CC, Faucett AN, et al. Automated real-time collection of pathogen-specific diagnostic data: syndromic infectious disease epidemiology. JMIR Public Health Surveill 2018;4(3):e59.
4. Benirschke RC, McElvania E, Thomson R, et al. Clinical impact of rapid point-of-care PCR influenza testing in an urgent care setting: a single-center study. J Clin Microbiol 2019;57(3) [pii:e01281-18].
5. Brachmann M, Kikull K, Kill C, et al. Economic and operational impact of an improved pathway using rapid molecular diagnostic testing for patients with influenza-like illness in a German emergency department. J Clin Monit Comput 2019. [Epub ahead of print].
6. Pang X, Lee BE. Laboratory diagnosis of noroviruses: present and future. Clin Lab Med 2015;35(2):345–62.
7. Buss SN, Alter R, Iwen PC, et al. Implications of culture-independent panel-based detection of Cyclospora cayetanensis. J Clin Microbiol 2013;51(11):3909.
8. Shane AL, Mody RK, Crump JA, et al. 2017 infectious diseases Society of America clinical practice guidelines for the diagnosis and management of infectious diarrhea. Clin Infect Dis 2017;65(12):1963–73.
9. Atkinson R, Maguire H, Gerner-Smidt P. A challenge and an opportunity to improve patient management and public health surveillance for food-borne infections through culture-independent diagnostics. J Clin Microbiol 2013;51(8):2479–82.
10. Shea S, Kubota KA, Maguire H, et al. Clinical microbiology laboratories' adoption of culture-independent diagnostic tests is a threat to foodborne-disease surveillance in the United States. J Clin Microbiol 2017;55(1):10–9.

11. Imdad A, Retzer F, Thomas LS, et al. Impact of culture-independent diagnostic testing on recovery of enteric bacterial infections. Clin Infect Dis 2018;66(12): 1892–8.

12. Goldstein EJ. Anaerobic bacteremia. Clin Infect Dis 1996;23(Suppl 1):S97–101.

13. Sinha M, Jupe J, Mack H, et al. Emerging technologies for molecular diagnosis of sepsis. Clin Microbiol Rev 2018;31(2).

14. Fraley SI, Hardick J, Masek BJ, et al. Universal digital high-resolution melt: a novel approach to broad-based profiling of heterogeneous biological samples. Nucleic Acids Res 2013;41(18):e175.

15. McHugh L, Seldon TA, Brandon RA, et al. A molecular host response assay to discriminate between sepsis and infection-negative systemic inflammation in critically ill patients: discovery and validation in independent cohorts. PLoS Med 2015;12(12):e1001916.

16. Zimmerman JJ, Sullivan E, Yager TD, et al. Diagnostic accuracy of a host gene expression signature that discriminates clinical severe sepsis syndrome and infection-negative systemic inflammation among critically ill children. Crit Care Med 2017;45(4):e418–25.

17. Sulaiman T, Salazar L, Hasbun R. Acute versus subacute community-acquired meningitis: analysis of 611 patients. Medicine (Baltimore) 2017;96(36):e7984.

18. Gutierrez-Murgas Y, Snowden JN. Ventricular shunt infections: immunopathogenesis and clinical management. J Neuroimmunol 2014;276(1–2):1–8.

19. Banks JT, Bharara S, Tubbs RS, et al. Polymerase chain reaction for the rapid detection of cerebrospinal fluid shunt or ventriculostomy infections. Neurosurgery 2005;57(6):1237–43 [discussion: 1237–43].

20. Busch MP, Kleinman SH, Tobler LH, et al. Virus and antibody dynamics in acute west Nile virus infection. J Infect Dis 2008;198(7):984–93.

21. Lustig Y, Mannasse B, Koren R, et al. Superiority of West Nile virus RNA detection in whole blood for diagnosis of acute infection. J Clin Microbiol 2016;54(9): 2294–7.

22. Barzon L, Pacenti M, Franchin E, et al. Excretion of West Nile virus in urine during acute infection. J Infect Dis 2013;208(7):1086–92.

23. Ferreira JE, Ferreira SC, Almeida-Neto C, et al. Molecular characterization of viruses associated with encephalitis in Sao Paulo, Brazil. PLoS One 2019;14(1): e0209993.

24. Sakushima K, Hayashino Y, Kawaguchi T, et al. Diagnostic accuracy of cerebrospinal fluid lactate for differentiating bacterial meningitis from aseptic meningitis: a meta-analysis. J Infect 2011;62(4):255–62.

25. Fortuna D, Hooper DC, Roberts AL, et al. Potential role of CSF cytokine profiles in discriminating infectious from non-infectious CNS disorders. PLoS One 2018; 13(10):e0205501.

26. Tristram S, Jacobs MR, Appelbaum PC. Antimicrobial resistance in Haemophilus influenzae. Clin Microbiol Rev 2007;20(2):368–89.

Predicting Bacterial Versus Viral Infection, or None of the Above

Current and Future Prospects of Biomarkers

Stefan Riedel, MD, PhD, D(ABMM)

KEYWORDS

- Biomarkers • Procalcitonin • Proadrenomedulin • C-reactive protein • Lactate
- Sepsis • Pneumonia • Antimicrobial stewardship

KEY POINTS

- Known and emerging infectious diseases, including sepsis and pneumonia, remain significant medical problems worldwide, and will continue to provide diagnostic challenges to physicians and laboratorians.
- Despite the availability of numerous biomarkers, no single biomarker has yet shown consistently high diagnostic and prognostic accuracy for sepsis, pneumonia, or other infectious diseases.
- The best evidence in support of diagnostic and prognostic utility in the management of patients with sepsis and pneumonia exists for the following traditional biomarkers: procalcitonin, C-reactive protein, and proadrenomedullin.
- The use of biomarker panels has shown improved diagnostic and prognostic performance characteristics compared with the use of a single biomarker alone.
- Integration of traditional pathogen-identification methods in microbiology, traditional biomarkers (eg, procalcitonin, proadrenomedullin), and emerging technologies (eg, proteomics, metabolomics) into complex algorithms is likely to improve the diagnosis and management of various infectious diseases in the near future.

INTRODUCTION

Despite many advances in diagnosis and treatment, infectious diseases remain a major cause of morbidity and mortality, worldwide. According to the US Centers for Disease Control and Prevention (CDC) in 2016, influenza and pneumonia were the eighth

Disclosure: S. Riedel has received research funding in the past from B.R.A.H.M.S. AG, Henningsdorf, Germany and Thermo Fisher Scientific, Middletown, VA.
Department of Pathology, Beth Israel Deaconess Medical Center, Harvard Medical School, 330 Brookline Avenue, Yamins 309, Boston, MA 02215, USA
E-mail address: sriedel@bidmc.harvard.edu

leading cause of death in the United States, closely followed by septicemia.[1] Sepsis has repeatedly been recognized globally as an important medical problem with significant morbidity and mortality,[2–4] and on May 26, 2017, the World Health Assembly, the World Health Organization's decision-making body, adopted a resolution on improving the prevention, diagnosis, and management of sepsis.[5] Acute febrile illness (AFI) is one of the most common reasons for patients to seek medical care either in the primary care setting or the emergency department (ED).[6] Because AFI may have both infectious and noninfectious causes, establishing an accurate diagnosis of a potentially severe infection (eg, sepsis or bacterial pneumonia) is often challenging to health care providers in acute clinical care settings. Furthermore, many, if not all, infectious diseases have the potential to ultimately result in life-threatening conditions; early recognition, assessment of severity, and rapid detection of the causative microorganism are critical for establishing the appropriate antimicrobial therapy.[7,8]

The clinical signs and symptoms of infections are a reflection of a dysregulated host immune response following the invasion of the host by a pathogenic infectious microorganism.[9] This immunologic host response is typically initiated by the recognition of pathogen-associated molecular patterns (PAMPs) from invasive microorganisms by the cells of the innate immune system.[9,10] The various cells of the innate immune system have pattern-recognition receptors, such as Toll-like receptors (TLRs) or nucleotide-binding oligomerization domain–like (NOD-like) receptors (NLRs), which are capable of recognizing PAMPs from various pathogenic microorganisms (eg, bacteria, viruses, fungi).[9,10] In addition, the pattern-recognition receptors on cells of the innate immune system are also capable of recognizing endogenous, danger-associated molecular patterns that are released during inflammatory stress and tissue damage (eg, burns, trauma, tissue necrosis).[10] When engaged by microbial ligands, TLRs and/or NLRs on macrophages result in the upregulation and release of proinflammatory cytokines, namely tumor necrosis factor (TNF), interleukin (IL)-1β, and IL-6.[9,11,12] These proinflammatory cytokines are mainly responsible for the upregulation and release of various proteins known as acute phase reactants (eg, C-reactive protein [CRP], procalcitonin [PCT]), the activation of endothelial cells, and the attraction of circulating polymorphonuclear leukocytes to the site of the infection. In addition, chemotactic cytokines (IL-8, monocyte chemoattractant protein [MCP-1], complement cascade proteins, biomarkers of activated neutrophils [eg, CD64, triggering receptor expressed on myeloid cells-1 (TREM-1), soluble TREM-1 (sTREM-1)], biomarkers of the antiinflammatory phase, as well as biomarkers of organ dysfunction [eg, lactate]) have been part of the complex host response to specific infectious disease states.[11,12] The discussion of the individual components of the innate immune response to infection and inflammation is beyond the scope of this article; interested readers are referred to the pertinent literature on this topic.

From a clinical perspective, physiologic changes in a patient's response to infection (eg, changes in body temperature, heart rate, respiratory rate, and leukocyte count) have long been used as diagnostic and prognostic indicators of infections, and are specifically components of algorithms for the diagnosis of sepsis and/or pneumonia.[13,14] These criteria are otherwise known as systemic inflammatory response syndrome (SIRS), and were part of the earlier Consensus Definitions for Sepsis and Septic Shock (**Table 1**).[13] Recognizing the complexity of the pathophysiology of sepsis, the Society of Critical Care Medicine and the European Society of Intensive Care Medicine convened a task force in 2014, in order to reevaluate the original guidelines. The task force sought to differentiate sepsis from other (uncomplicated) infections, in which some SIRS criteria might be present, and new, updated guidelines for sepsis and septic shock were published in 2016 (Sepsis-3), defining sepsis now

Table 1 Systemic inflammatory response syndrome criteria	
Temperature	>38°C or <36°C
Heart Rate	>90/min
Respiratory Rate	>20/min or $Paco_2$ <4.3 kPa
Leukocyte Count	>12,000/μL or <4000/μL

Two or more SIRS criteria in addition to a blood culture–confirmed bloodstream infection are considered to indicate sepsis.
Data from Bone RC, Balk RA, Cerra FB, et al. Definitions for sepsis and organ failure and guidelines for the use of innovative therapies in sepsis. The ACCP/SCCM Consensus Conference Committee. American College of Chest Physicians/Society of Critical Care Medicine. Crit Care Med 1992;20(6):864–74.

as a life-threatening organ dysfunction caused by a dysregulated host response to infection.[3] In addition to SIRS criteria, clinical diagnostic criteria, namely the Sequential Organ Failure Assessment (SOFA), and the Quick SOFA (qSOFA) scores for sepsis and septic shock, were included in the updated diagnostic guidelines, mainly for intensive care unit (ICU) patients.[3] However, the clinical scoring systems are not intended as stand-alone criteria for sepsis, and the task force emphasized that SIRS criteria still remain useful in the assessment of febrile patients for the identification of infection. As with sepsis, appropriate initial severity assessment is a critical step in the management of pneumonia, and guidelines for the diagnosis and management of community-acquired pneumonia (CAP), health care–associated pneumonia, and ventilator-associated pneumonia have emphasized the utility of various clinical scoring systems (eg, Clinical Pulmonary Infection Score, pneumonia severity index [PSI], and SOFA) for early recognition and implementation of appropriate antimicrobial therapy.[15–19]

Although these various clinical scoring systems have shown a tremendous benefit for the rapid clinical assessment of patients suspected to have pneumonia and/or sepsis, they have only moderate prognostic accuracy and were validated for mortality assessment only. Furthermore, clinical microbiology laboratory tests remain essential components for the diagnosis of infectious diseases.[20–22] In sepsis and pneumonia, the ultimate proof of the infection is provided by obtaining a blood culture (BC) and/or sputum culture, respectively, that is positive for bacterial and/or fungal organisms.[3,15,21,22] However, the culture-based confirmation of an infection is only an imperfect gold standard. For example, in patients with pneumonia, antimicrobial therapy is often implemented before laboratory specimens for bacteriologic culture have been obtained, therefore potentially compromising the isolation of the bacterial cause of the infection. Various studies have shown that BCs, despite being considered the gold standard for the confirmation of sepsis, are positive in only some 50% of all cases.[23–25] Furthermore, culture-based methods do not provide rapid organism detection because of the time required for organisms to grow on specific media, and therefore have longer turn-around times (TATs) for results, including the additional antimicrobial susceptibility testing (AST).[22] Therefore, such diagnostic limitations are commonly compensated for by the liberal use of broad-spectrum antimicrobial therapy. However, at times of globally increasing antimicrobial resistance in both gram-positive and gram-negative organisms, antimicrobial stewardship programs are working to decrease such potential overuse of broad-spectrum antimicrobial agents. In addition, there is a continued and growing interest to develop more diagnostic and/or prognostic laboratory tests with shorter TATs to assist in the management of critically ill patients with infections.

THE ROLE OF BIOMARKERS IN DIAGNOSIS AND MANAGEMENT OF INFECTIOUS DISEASES

Biomarkers have been defined as analytes that can be objectively measured and evaluated to assess a normal physiologic or pathologic process, or the response to a pharmacologic/therapeutic intervention.[26] In order to be considered clinical useful, a biomarker should meet most if not all of the following prerequisite characteristics: accurate reflection of a physiologic or pathophysiologic state or process; appropriately high sensitivity and specificity; high positive predictive value and negative predictive value; diagnostic accuracy as assessed by calculation of positive and negative likelihood ratios.[26,27] However, an absolute and accurate assessment of the clinical utility of any biomarker is difficult to achieve, considering that there is a tremendous variation of laboratory assays and methodologies, as well as the chosen cutoff values between the many published clinical and/or laboratory-based studies. In addition, any biomarker assay in the laboratory should also be readily available for clinicians to order, and have a short TAT, in order to be considered clinically useful.[28] **Table 2** provides an overview of the biomarkers that are most commonly used in sepsis, lower respiratory tract infections (LRTIs), and other infectious diseases, and that are discussed in more detail later.

In general, biomarkers can be divided into 2 categories: diagnostic and prognostic. However, some biomarkers may fulfill both criteria. Recognizing the limitations of clinical scoring systems as well as standard, culture-based laboratory tests for organism identification and AST, the need for biomarker testing to assess the immunologic host response to infection has long been recognized as a valuable asset to improving the diagnosis of infectious diseases and to providing prognostic information to aid in the implementation of the most appropriate therapeutic interventions. During the last 2 decades, interest in identifying biomarkers for the diagnosis of sepsis and other infectious diseases has gained a significantly greater momentum. Although more than 100 biomarkers for inflammation and infectious diseases have been identified, only a few biomarkers have been repeatedly included in numerous studies and shown some utility in the diagnosis and management of key infectious diseases such as sepsis and pneumonia.[28] These biomarkers include CRP, PCT, and lactate. Using the approach of a crude PubMed database search for publications including the keywords "(infection *or* sepsis *or* pneumonia) *and* biomarkers," more than 30,000 articles were identified that have been published within the last 20 years. More specifically, within this same time frame, more than 5000 articles were published on biomarkers in sepsis and slightly more than 2000 articles were published on biomarkers in pneumonia (**Fig. 1**A, B). A large number of these publications are focused investigations of PCT in sepsis and/or pneumonia (**Fig. 2**A, B). In addition, at the time of writing this article, 143 clinical trials are active and/or enrolling patients into studies investigating the role of biomarkers in sepsis[29]; 122 clinical trials are registered and actively enrolling patients into studies investigating the role of biomarkers in pneumonia.[30] Despite the magnitude of publications and the continued interest in biomarkers for infectious diseases, so far, no individual biomarker has been identified to reliably diagnose sepsis and/or bacterial pneumonia. However, a few biomarkers, and PCT in particular, have shown higher levels of performance, often in combination with other clinical and/or laboratory data for providing diagnostic and prognostic information for patients with sepsis and pneumonia. This article next addresses specific biomarkers that have

Table 2
Role of biomarkers in infectious disease diagnostics, identified by literature search, with select references

Biomarker Test	Commercially Available	Patient Population		Biomarker Has Utility in Sepsis		Biomarker Has Utility in LRTI		Evaluated for Other Clinical Indications	Usefulness for Support of Antimicrobial Stewardship	Specific Considerations	References
		Adult	Pediatric	Diagnostic	Prognostic	Diagnostic	Prognostic				
PCT	Yes[a]	X	X	Yes	Yes	Yes	Yes	Meningitis; urinary tract infection; COPD exacerbation	Yes	High sensitivity and specificity; useful for differentiation between bacterial and viral infections	6,37,46, 53–76,92, 94,100
Pro-ADM	Yes[b]	X	X	No	Yes	No	Yes	—	Probable	Limited data on antimicrobial stewardship support	6,37,68, 77–85, 100
CRP	Yes[a]	X	X	Yes	Unclear	Yes	Limited	Numerous infections and inflammatory conditions	No/limited	Low specificity	6,33–39, 68,92, 94,100
PTX3	No	X	—	Probable	Probable	No	No	Tuberculosis; meningitis; viral infections, incl. Influenza	—	—	6,37,41–45, 68,100
Presepsin	No	X	—	Yes	Yes	Unclear	Unclear	—	No	High specificity	6,98–100
sTREM-1	No	X	—	Probable	Probable	Probable	Probable	—	—	Limited clinical data available	6,96,97,100
IL-6/IL-8	Yes[b]	X	X	Yes, weak	Yes, weak	Unclear	Unclear	—	—	—	6,37,91–94
Lactate	Yes[a]	X	X	No	Yes	No	No	—	No	—	68,86–90

X, studies met specific criteria and patient care settings for which the biomarker was evaluated; —, criteria not applicable or not evaluated, no data available.
Abbreviations: COPD, chronic obstructive pulmonary disease; CRP, C-reactive protein; IL, interleukin; LRTI, lower respiratory tract infection, including pneumonia; PCT, procalcitonin; pro-ADM, proadrenomedullin; PTX3, pentraxin 3; sTREM-1, soluble triggering receptor expressed on myeloid cells-1.
a US Food and Drug Administration (FDA) cleared for this indication and assays are FDA cleared for clinical use.
b Not FDA cleared for this clinical indication and/or assay is not FDA approved for clinical use.

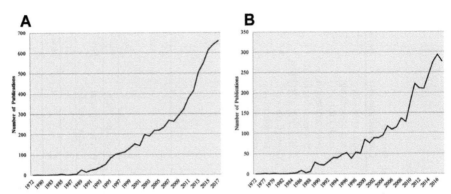

Fig. 1. (*A*) Articles published and indexed in the PubMed database, with the search term "sepsis AND biomarkers" between 1972 and 2017. (*B*) Articles published and indexed in the PubMed database, with the search term "pneumonia AND biomarkers" between 1972 and 2017.

shown clinical utility for the diagnosis and management of these 2 clinical infectious entities. It then describes the potential future directions for biomarkers and other diagnostic modalities in support of diagnosis and prognosis of infectious diseases.

The Role of Biomarkers for the Diagnosis and Management of Sepsis

Among the more than 100 biomarkers studied for sepsis, there are only a few biomarkers that have consistently shown good diagnostic and/or prognostic value.[28] A recent, retrospective, observational study investigated the "real-world use of procalcitonin and other biomarkers among sepsis hospitalizations in the United States."[31] Using data from the Premier Healthcare Database (including more than 700 US hospitals), the investigators found that, during a 3-year period, among 933,591 patients with identified septicemia, 78% had biomarker tests ordered during their course of hospitalization. Although severity of illness was a common thread in the use of biomarkers, the use of lactate and CRP remained constant over time, whereas a 6-fold increase in use of PCT was observed, reflecting the continued and increasing interest in biomarkers for the diagnosis and prognosis of sepsis.[31] The following key biomarkers have consistently been shown to have clinical utility and are subject to

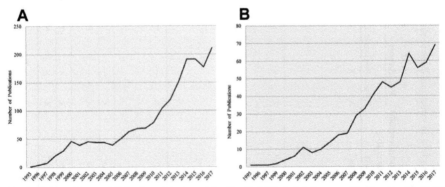

Fig. 2. (*A*) Articles published and indexed in the PubMed database, with the search term "sepsis AND procalcitonin" between 1993 and 2017. (*B*) Articles published and indexed in the PubMed database, with the search term "pneumonia AND procalcitonin" between 1995 and 2017.

many past and ongoing studies: CRP, pentraxin-3 (PTX3), PCT, IL-6, IL-8, proadreno-medullin (pro-ADM), lactate, presepsin, and triggering receptor expressed on myeloid cells-1 (TREM-1).

C-reactive Protein

CRP is a well-established biomarker of inflammation and infection, and belongs to the pentraxin family of acute phase reactants.[32] CRP is synthesized primarily in the liver in response to cytokine stimulation (specifically IL-6 and IL-1β); protein secretion begins typically 4 to 6 hours after stimulation and peaks around 36 to 48 hours. Its half-life is approximately 19 hours. CRP binds to teichoic acid components in gram-positive bacteria, and to lipopolysaccharides in gram-negative bacteria.[33,34] Despite its low specificity for sepsis or any other infectious disease conditions, CRP continues to be commonly used to screen for early-onset sepsis. Although numerous studies suggest that perhaps even a single increased CRP value together with other clinical indicators may support the suspicion of sepsis, other studies identified the limitations of this biomarker as a diagnostic as well as prognostic tool, specifically in critically ill patients (eg, ICU setting), when other inflammatory conditions and comorbidities are present.[34–37] As with its limitation as a diagnostic marker, a single CRP level has also shown to have limited prognostic value; however, serial CRP assessments have been shown in various studies to be of prognostic value when assessing morbidity and mortality of patients with sepsis progressing to severe sepsis; in addition, some studies suggest that CRP is a good marker to predict the response to antimicrobial therapy.[38,39]

Pentraxin-3

PTX3 belongs to the subfamily of so-called long pentraxins, which are acute phase proteins that act as pattern-recognition receptors in acute immunologic responses (including the humoral innate immune response) to microbial infections.[39–41] PTX3 is secreted by multiple cells, including dendritic cells, monocytes, neutrophils, endothelial cells, and epithelial cells, in response to stimulation by cytokines such as IL-1, TNF-α, and TLRs; however, IL-6 and interferons do not result in PTX3 secretion.[41] Various specific microorganisms have been shown to cause increased PTX3 expression: *Staphylococcus aureus, Pseudomonas aeruginosa, Klebsiella pneumoniae, Escherichia coli, Neisseria meningitides*, as well as *Aspergillus fumigatus*.[41] In addition several viruses, including influenza virus A, can also lead to PTX3 upregulation and secretion.[41] The PTX3 plasma concentration in healthy individuals is barely detectable (<2 ng/mL); however, concentrations significantly increase rapidly within 6 to 8 hours (>100 ng/mL) during severe sepsis and septic shock.[40,41] One study showed that increased levels of PTX3 in patients with severe sepsis and septic shock remained significantly higher during the first week of sepsis in nonsurvivors compared with survivors.[42] In another recent study, the investigators showed that PTX3 is useful in discriminating the various stages of sepsis according to the sepsis-3 definitions.[43] Specifically, measurements of PTX3 on days 1, 3, and 8 of ICU admission reliably differentiated between sepsis, severe sepsis, and septic shock; furthermore, PTX3 accurately correlated with assessment of disease severity and organ dysfunction compared with clinical scoring systems (eg, SOFA).[43] Two studies showed the value of PTX3 measurements in patients presenting to the ED with signs/symptoms of sepsis.[44,45] Both studies showed the ability of PTX3 to aid in the diagnosis of sepsis, and furthermore to stratify patients according to severity of sepsis and prediction of mortality. Furthermore, PTX3 had positive correlation with other biomarkers, such as PCT and CRP, in addition to clinical scoring systems.[45] The study by

Uusitalo-Seppälä and colleagues[45] showed that high levels of PCT and PTX3 are useful as prognostic markers in patients with sepsis presenting to the ED and are independent predictors of progression to severe sepsis and mortality. In addition to its utility as a diagnostic and prognostic marker in sepsis, increased levels of PTX3 have also been shown in other infectious diseases, such as pulmonary tuberculosis, meningococcal disease, and dengue fever.[41] However, additional studies, including multicenter, randomized trials, will be necessary to further investigate the utility of PTX3 in infections other than sepsis and pneumonia.

Procalcitonin

By far the most studied biomarker during the past 10 years has been PCT, which has shown both diagnostic and prognostic utilities. PCT is a member of the *CAPA* protein family, and a precursor peptide for the hormone calcitonin.[46] In its main role to maintain calcium homeostasis, calcitonin also inhibits osteoclast activity and therefore prevents bone resorption. In 1993, Assicot and colleagues[47] first recognized that PCT levels in serum were significantly increased in patients with sepsis and microbial infections, as well as severe inflammatory conditions. In bacterial infections, the production of PCT is upregulated by the organisms' toxins as well as by proinflammatory mediators (eg, IL-1, TNF-α, and IL-6), whereas the increase of interferon-γ during viral infections inhibits the production and release of PCT.[48] In healthy individuals, and in the absence of systemic bacterial infections, PCT levels are low ($\leq$0.1 ng/mL) and its release is restricted to the neuroendocrine C cells of the thyroid gland; however, the expression and release of PCT are upregulated during sepsis and other systemic infections, and PCT is constitutively released from nearly all tissues and cell types in the body.[49] During systemic bacterial infections, such as sepsis, PCT levels increase within 3 to 6 hours of the onset of the infection.[50,51] Serum levels peak at 12 to 24 hours; the half-life of PCT is 24 hours, and, on cessation of the infection, PCT levels typically decrease by 50% per day.[50,51] However, in uncontrolled and continuing infections, PCT levels remain increased and may even continue to increase. This favorable kinetic profile of PCT, its rapid increase, sustainment during infection, and decrease during appropriate antimicrobial therapy make it an ideal diagnostic and prognostic biomarker. In addition, it is noteworthy that PCT levels, compared with those of other biomarkers (eg, CRP), remain unaffected in neutropenic patients or by the administration of immunosuppressive therapy (eg, corticosteroids).[52] Several studies have shown that increasing PCT levels are useful in diagnosing sepsis.[53–58] Data from a multicenter cohort study showed that initial PCT levels in the ED accurately predict BC positivity in patients with CAP.[53] Other studies found that PCT is a valuable diagnostic biomarker for sepsis in febrile patients presenting to the ED.[54,55] In one setting, the combination of PCT with clinical scoring criteria significantly enhanced the value of diagnostic algorithms for sepsis,[54] whereas in the other study, the investigators showed that bacteria and/or sepsis are unlikely to be present at PCT levels of less than or equal to 1 ng/mL.[55] Other studies compared the diagnostic utility of PCT with that of other biomarkers, including CRP. In a study of 3343 patients suspected to have sepsis, BC results were compared with PCT and CRP levels; the investigators found that PCT levels in patients with bacteremia/sepsis were significantly higher compared with patients without bacteremia ($P<.0001$).[56] Furthermore, PCT was found to be a more reliable marker for prediction of bacteremia compared with CRP. In addition, the investigators found that median PCT concentrations in patients with gram-negative sepsis (5.0 ng/mL) were statistically significantly higher ($P = .0003$) compared with median PCT levels in gram-positive sepsis (2.0 ng/mL) and/or fungemia (2.1 ng/mL).[56] Similar results were described in 2 more recent studies investigating the utility of PCT and CRP in patients with gram-positive and gram-negative sepsis, whereby patients with gram-negative sepsis presented with significantly higher levels of PCT compared with patients with gram-positive sepsis.[57,58] In addition, PCT has also been useful in patients with positive BCs and suspected to have sepsis to differentiate between BC contaminants and organisms representing true bacteremia.[59] Furthermore, PCT has proved to be a useful and sensitive biomarker for the diagnosis of bacteremia/sepsis in children as well as elderly patients.[60,61] Several meta-analyses have been performed on the diagnostic accuracy of PCT.[62–66] Four of these meta-analyses identified PCT as a useful biomarker with at least good performance for the diagnosis of sepsis,[63–66] whereas 1 meta-analysis identified only a moderate benefit in the detection of bacteremia/sepsis.[62] In a recent meta-analysis for the utility of PCT in neonatal sepsis and children with SIRS, the investigators found that PCT has moderate accuracy for the diagnosis of sepsis in neonates when using a cutoff value of 2.0 to 2.5 ng/mL.[67] Based on the cumulative evidence presented here, PCT can safely be considered a valuable diagnostic biomarker, and serum levels between 0.1 ng/mL and 0.5 ng/mL suggest the presence of bacterial infection for which antimicrobial therapy would be required; however, no consensus has been reached on the definitive cutoff value for PCT in this decision process.[66] In addition to its diagnostic role in sepsis, PCT has also been shown to be a useful prognostic test to aid in the management of patients with sepsis.[68–75] Although 1 earlier study showed that PCT levels increase with increasing severity of sepsis and associated organ dysfunction,[69] in another study PCT failed to show such predictive characteristics.[69] Subsequent studies, from small, proof-of-concept studies to randomized, multicenter studies, found that PCT-guided antibiotic therapy in patients in the ED and ICU can safely lead to reduction of (unnecessary) antimicrobial therapy.[70–73] More recently, a prospective observational study, enrolling 858 patients with sepsis, showed that the lack of decreasing PCT levels by greater than 80% between baseline and day 4 was associated with a significantly higher mortality.[74] Although there was a 2-fold higher risk of death for patients with a decrease in PCT less than or equal to 80%, compared with those with greater than 80% decrease in the first 4 days following ICU admission, a baseline PCT of greater than 2.0 ng/mL was an additional risk factor and associated with at least a 3-fold greater mortality risk.[74] A recent, patient-level meta-analysis of 11 clinical, randomized trials investigated the impact of PCT-guided antimicrobial therapy on mortality of ICU patients with infection and sepsis.[75] The investigators found that mortality in 2252 patients with PCT-guided therapy was significantly lower compared with the 2230 patients in the control group.[75] A further subgroup analysis stratified by the type of infections present (eg, sepsis, pneumonia, urinary tract infection) confirmed the overall effects on reduction of mortality.[75] Two recent, retrospective, observational, cohort studies investigated the "real-world use of procalcitonin and other biomarkers among sepsis hospitalizations in the United States."[31,76] Using data from the Premier Healthcare Database, both studies performed regression analyses to assess the association of PCT use and outcomes for patients with sepsis and other infections in the United States. These studies have contradicting results with regard to the impact of PCT use and PCT-guided antimicrobial use on mortality. Although the study by Chu and colleagues[76] found that PCT was not associated with decreased mortality, the study by Gluck and colleagues[31] concluded that PCT use was associated with decreased in-hospital mortality. These differences could be explained by the differences in study duration (1 year vs 3 years) and the study by Chu and colleagues[76] did not include an adjustment for severity of illness in the analyses. In addition, both studies did not observe an association between PCT testing and antimicrobial use.[31,76] However, both studies underscore that there is an increasing need for biomarker testing (including use of PCT) as a component for the diagnosis and management of sepsis.

Proadrenomedullin

Adrenomedullin and pro-ADM are biomarkers related to the regulation of the vasotonus, and have been shown to contribute to the multitude of hemodynamic alterations during sepsis, and specifically during the earl phases of severe sepsis.[37] ADM is a vasodilative biomarker, showing both natriuretic and diuretic properties.[77] Initially identified in pheochromocytoma, levels of ADM and its midregional amino acid sequence pro-ADM were subsequently shown to be increased in patients with sepsis.[78] In numerous subsequent studies, pro-ADM was shown to be an excellent prognostic biomarker for assessment of severity and outcome of sepsis.[79–84] In a prospective, observational study of 101 patients with SIRS and sepsis, severe sepsis, and/or septic shock, pro-ADM showed excellent prognostic utility, which was equal to or better than clinical scoring systems and superior to other biomarkers that were included in the study (PCT, CRP, IL-6).[79] Other, more recent studies showed that pro-ADM, alone or in combination with biomarkers such as PCT, has excellent performance characteristics for the prognosis of sepsis.[80–83] In a study of 99 ICU patients with septic shock, both pro-vasopressin (pro-AVP) and pro-ADM serum concentrations were significantly higher in nonsurvivors compared with survivors, and therefore were found to be good predictors of 28-day mortality.[80] Similarly, in a single-center study with 114 critically ill, febrile patients with cancer, 27 patients were identified to have sepsis and compared with those with localized infections and no infections.[81] Pro-ADM and PCT were better diagnostic markers of bloodstream infection/sepsis compared with CRP; similarly, both biomarkers were superior to CRP as predictors of the response to antimicrobial therapy; however, pro-ADM was a better prognostic marker than PCT.[81]

In a more recent study of 1089 ICU patients with sepsis, pro-ADM identified disease severity and treatment response more accurately than other biomarkers and clinical scoring systems.[82] Using clinical scores as a comparator, one study showed that the performance of pro-ADM and other biomarkers in predicting mortality in sepsis depends strongly on the degree of organ failure present on ICU admission.[84] However, pro-ADM was the only biomarker that reliably identified nonsurvivors across all severity groups of patients.[84] In addition, a recent meta-analysis confirmed data from these various prior, often single-center studies, showing that pro-ADM is a clinically useful biomarker for the prediction of mortality risk in patients with sepsis.[85]

Additional Biomarkers for Sepsis

Numerous other sepsis biomarkers have been studied in various settings during the past 2 decades; however, it is beyond the scope of this article to provide a comprehensive review of all markers. A few examples of additional, well-studied biomarkers in sepsis include IL-6, IL-8, lactate, and sTREM-1. For many decades, lactate has been widely used as a diagnostic and prognostic biomarker for sepsis in patients in the ED as well as the ICU settings, and the sepsis-3 definition includes lactate levels in the definition of septic shock.[3] The association between increased lactate levels and mortality has been established in several studies.[86–88] Lactate levels greater than 4 mmol/L have shown a particularly strong association with increased mortality.[86] In addition, serial lactate measurements may be useful in monitoring treatment efficacy and continue to be recommended as part of the sepsis guidelines.[3,14] Despite lactate being a commonly used analyte to monitor patients with sepsis, this marker does present several limitations. Increased lactate levels have been described in several conditions other than sepsis, including cardiogenic shock, trauma, seizure, intoxications, burns, and diabetic ketoacidosis.[89] Furthermore, although normal lactate levels are often interpreted as indicators for a good prognosis, some studies found that normal lactate levels in patients with sepsis may still be associated with an increased mortality risk. For example, one study found that 45% of patients with vasopressor-dependent septic shock and associated lactate levels of less than 2.4 mmol/L still have an associated mortality of 20%.[90] Although lactate is a well-established and supported prognostic marker for the assessment of severe sepsis and septic shock, it should not be used as a stand-alone test for the diagnosis and management of sepsis, but should be interpreted in the context of clinical patient assessment and other laboratory markers.[3,12]

Cytokines are the major contributors to the various pathophysiologic processes across the spectrum of sepsis.[9–11] Two cytokines, namely IL-6 and IL-8, have repeatedly been included in studies investigating sepsis biomarkers; because of the high variability of sensitivity and specificity found in many studies, none of the cytokines are currently used in routine clinical practice. IL-6 was first proposed as a biomarker for early sepsis diagnosis in neonates presenting to the ED.[91,92] One study proposed the use of cytokine profiles rather than the use of a single cytokine as a marker of sepsis.[93] This study showed that the proinflammatory cytokines IL-6 and IL-8, as well as the immunosuppressive cytokine IL-10, had higher serum concentrations during the early stages of sepsis in patients with ultimately fatal outcomes, compared with survivors.[93] In earlier studies, IL-6 showed some utility as a predictor of early-onset sepsis because its levels typically peak during the first 48 hours of sepsis.[94] However, based on currently available data from studies, all of which are limited by the number of enrolled patients, the sensitivity of cytokines, specifically IL-6, as sepsis biomarkers depends on the chosen cutoff value, and for neonatal sepsis gestational age–dependent level should be taken into consideration as well.[91] The specificity for IL-8 in these studies was similar to the specificity for IL-6; however, the corresponding mean sensitivities were slightly lower.[37,93]

In addition, some other promising biomarkers for sepsis include markers expressed on the membranes of macrophages and monocytes: sTREM, presepsin (CD14), and CD64.[12,37] TREM-1, like CD64, is located on the surface of mature monocytes and polymorphonuclear neutrophils; its expression increases in the setting of bacterial infections, and its soluble form is released into the serum.[95] Despite a recent meta-analysis assessing the clinical utility of sTREM-1 for diagnosis of sepsis finding that this marker had only a moderate diagnostic performance for differentiating sepsis from SIRS,[96] several other studies found increased levels of sTREM-1 in various infectious diseases and other clinical settings, suggesting that sTREM-1 may eventually be a useful biomarker in diagnostic algorithms for sepsis and other infectious diseases.[97] Presepsin is the soluble form of CD14, which is expressed on the membranes of myeloid cells and monocytes.[98] Although its physiologic role has not been fully established yet, increased presepsin levels have been identified during early stages of gram-positive and gram-negative sepsis.[98] One study suggested that the diagnostic utility of presepsin is comparable with that of PCT, and correlated with severity of illness.[99] This biomarker showed high specificity, and the results from clinical as well as experimental studies have been encouraging, supporting the need for further, more comprehensive clinical studies.[100]

The Role of Biomarkers for the Diagnosis and Management of Pneumonia

According to the CDC, LRTIs, specifically bacterial pneumonia and influenza, are among the top 10 leading causes of death in the United States.[1,15] Although the diagnosis of pneumonia is still based on abnormal radiologic findings and clinical signs/symptoms (eg, fever; purulent sputum), several of the previously mentioned bio-markers have been evaluated as potential diagnostic and prognostic tests for pneumonia. Among those biomarkers, PCT has shown the most promising results for the diagnosis of pneumonia and furthermore differentiating bacterial from viral infection.[101] Compared with CRP and various cytokines, PCT had a higher sensitivity and accuracy for differentiation of bacterial pneumonia from viral infections.[101–103] Another study, comparing the utility of PCT and CRP for the diagnosis of CAP, found that increased PCT levels (>0.5 ng/mL) were a good indicator of bacterial pneumonia, specifically for invasive pneumococcal pneumonia.[104] However, the results from this study only supported PCT as being supplementary to clinical scoring systems (eg, PSI) for the assessment of disease severity.[104] With respect to severity assessment in CAP, pro-ADM has been shown to be of better prognostic value than PCT and other biomarkers.[105] A recent systematic review and meta-analysis analyzed data from 12 published studies investigating the prognostic utility of biomarkers and specifically pro-ADM in patients with CAP.[106] Based on the analyses of these studies, the investigators concluded that increased level of pro-ADM on admission is associated with higher short-term mortality (odds ratio [OR] = 6.8; $P<.001$) and complications from CAP (OR = 5.0; $P<.001$).[106] The study further showed that use of pro-ADM is a valuable addition to current clinical scoring systems for assessment of CAP. Despite the promising results from this meta-analysis, the investigators concluded that, because of the overall low number of studies and the lack of studies assessing long-term complications of CAP in this meta-analysis, additional larger, multicenter studies are needed to evaluate the utility of pro-ADM and other biomarkers as prognostic markers in CAP.[106]

In addition, biomarkers, and PCT in particular, have been evaluated for their role in antimicrobial stewardship decisions for LRTIs. Most studies supporting the use of biomarkers for diagnosis, risk stratification, and antibiotic treatment decisions in pneumonia were conducted in Europe, specifically Germany and Switzerland.[16,73,74,101,107–109] For example, data from a multicenter trial in Switzerland showed that the use of PCT-guided antibiotic therapy, and specifically the decision to initiate antibiotic therapy, resulted in reduction of (unnecessary) antibiotic exposure without any increase in associated adverse effects on patient care.[107] Despite these promising data for PCT-guided antibiotic stewardship from various trials in European countries, a recent multicenter study in 14 US hospitals evaluating antibiotic use in patients with LRTIs found that the use of PCT in conjunction with antibiotic stewardship guidelines did not result in a decrease of antibiotic usage compared with antibiotic use in patients in the control arm (standard care without PCT).[110] A recent systematic review and meta-analysis with focus on studies investigating the use of PCT-guided antibiotic decisions versus standard-of-care antibiotic decisions found that use of PCT-guided antibiotic use protocols overall did not result in a decrease in short-term mortality.[111] However, within the subgroup of studies investigating the benefits of PCT-guided antibiotic cessation, this meta-analysis found that PCT-guided antibiotic cessation resulted in decreased duration of antibiotic usage and associated decreased mortality.[111] Within the subgroup of the mixed approach (initiation/cessation) to PCT-guided antibiotic therapy, there was no associated decrease in mortality, nor a reduction in hospital and/or ICU length of stay.[111]

In summary, as with sepsis, there is no single diagnostic biomarker for bacterial pneumonia; however, data support that PCT may be useful in addition to current and standard clinical diagnostic criteria to differentiate between bacterial and viral pneumonia, at least in certain subsets of patients. Furthermore, the use of various biomarkers, and PCT and pro-ADM in particular, could help stratify patients with pneumonia according to severity and need for hospitalization and/or ICU admission. Data on the use of PCT-guided antibiotic stewardship are less clear, and do not conclusively support decisions (initiation and/or cessation) of antibiotic treatment based on PCT values alone. Furthermore, studies have shown clearly that the use of PCT-guided antibiotic decision algorithms heavily depends on strict adherence and compliance with such guidelines by all health care providers in order to be effective.

FUTURE DIRECTIONS FOR THE ROLE OF BIOMARKERS IN DIAGNOSIS OF INFECTIOUS DISEASES

So far, this article has provided a review of various biomarkers that are currently available for clinical testing to aid in the diagnosis and management of sepsis and LRTIs. Among these biomarkers, PCT and pro-ADM have repeatedly shown superior performance characteristics and clinical utility as diagnostic and prognostic markers compared with other biomarkers, such as CRP, IL-6, IL-8, and sTREM-1. However, in many instances, the successful use of any biomarker, including PCT and pro-ADM, depends on their integration into clinical guidelines for diagnosis and treatment of specific infectious diseases (eg, sepsis, pneumonia) and the strict adherence to such guidelines by clinicians, as mentioned earlier in the detailed discussion of the many comprehensive, multicenter clinical trials as well as in meta-analyses. Although the diagnostic and prognostic utilities of biomarkers are consistently and most frequently investigated for sepsis and LRTIs, there are some studies investigating the role of biomarkers for other infectious diseases. PCT has been shown to have some, albeit limited, utility in supporting the diagnosis and prognosis of meningitis and urinary tract infections.[112–114] In addition, aside from the traditional biomarkers described in this article, the search for novel biomarkers continues, and several markers based on research in genomics, transcriptomics, proteomics, and metabolomics have been proposed.[115–117]

During the past 2 decades, several emerging new technologies have improved the TAT for diagnostics of infectious diseases; among those are mass spectrometry–based technologies and molecular technologies, such as polymerase chain reaction–based techniques and nucleic acid sequencing (next-generation sequencing) technologies.[115–117] Furthermore, omics-based approaches have provided additional insight into the pathogen-host interactions for various infectious diseases.[116] Studies investigating the regulation of gene expression during specific infectious diseases (eg, sepsis), pathogen-dependent associations, and host transcriptomic signatures for various pathogen-host interactions provided further insight into the complexity of these infectious diseases.[116] Another emerging area of research is attempting to correlate the host-specific and pathogen-specific aspects of certain infectious disease conditions (eg, sepsis) in the context of the microbiome.[116–118] Although these novel technologies are providing deeper insights into the complexity of various infectious diseases, certain limitations and challenges have to be considered, specifically when comparing results from various studies and clinical trials. Specifically, data regarding study design, importantly inclusion criteria and microbiology laboratory methods for pathogen identification and AST, are important factors influencing any further analyses of data obtained through omics-based technologies. Differences in the scaling up of sequencing methods, the biological samples used for diagnostic testing, and the methods used for bioinformatics and data analyses are additional challenging and/or potentially limiting factors for comparison of various omics-based studies of infectious diseases. However, modeling approaches for the analysis of the host-pathogen-microbiome interactions are currently still in development and have not been fully established.[118] However, the future integration of these rapidly evolving omics-based diagnostic technologies will continue to change and improve infectious disease diagnostics in the coming years.

SUMMARY

During the past 20 years, the clinical interest in using biomarkers to differentiate between infectious and noninfectious causes of fever, as well as the differentiation between bacterial and viral infections, has grown tremendously. Although there is no lack of clinical studies and meta-analyses investigating the role of various biomarkers for the diagnosis of sepsis, pneumonia, and other infectious diseases, it is clear that there is no single, ideal biomarker for the diagnosis of any single infectious disease. Nevertheless, a few biomarkers have repeatedly been shown to possess superior characteristics; among those are PCT and pro-ADM, which have repeatedly shown excellent performance characteristics for the diagnosis and prognosis of sepsis and LRTIs. Furthermore, the use of biomarker panels, including various combinations of those markers listed earlier, may have shown better performance characteristics compared with a single biomarker alone. There are a few fundamental limitations for establishing clinically useful biomarkers and biomarker panels that have to be considered. First and foremost, current limitations in the understanding of the complexities of the underlying pathophysiologic processes, including host-pathogen interactions, have to be considered when comparing the utility and impact on clinical outcomes of traditional biomarkers evaluated in the myriad of published studies. Furthermore, criteria for study inclusion as well as primary and other end points to measure the clinical impact and outcome also have to be considered. Future studies, including multicenter trials, will be necessary to continue the evaluation of clinical utility of traditional biomarkers. In addition, it is hoped that data derived from novel diagnostic and omics-based technologies will contribute to a better overall understanding of the underlying pathophysiologic processes of various infectious disease conditions. Furthermore, moving from a pathogen-focused approach for diagnostics to a comprehensive, pathobiome-based understanding of infections will require the inclusion of all diagnostic tests available: pathogen-identification methods, omics-based technologies for evaluation of the host-pathogen interaction, as well as traditional and emerging biomarkers reflecting the host response to a pathogen.

REFERENCES

1. Heron M. Deaths: leading causes for 2016. Natl Vital Stat Rep 2018;67(6):1–77.
2. Vincent J-L, Marshall JC, Namendys-Silva SA, et al. Assessment of the worldwide burden of critical illness: the Intensive Care over Nations (ICON) audit. Lancet Respir Med 2014;2(5):380–6.
3. Singer M, Deutschman CS, Seymour CW, et al. The third international consensus definitions for sepsis and septic shock (Sepsis-3). JAMA 2016; 315(8):801–10.
4. Rudd KE, Kissoon N, Limmathurotsakul D, et al. The global burden of sepsis: barriers and potential solutions. Crit Care 2018;22(1):232.
5. Reinhart K, Daniels R, Kissoon N, et al. Recognizing sepsis as a global health priority – A WHO Resolution. N Engl J Med 2017;377(5):414–7.
6. Kapasi AJ, Dittrich S, Gonzalez IJ, et al. Host biomarkers distinguishing bacterial from non-bacterial causes of acute febrile illness: a comprehensive review. PLoS One 2016;11(8):e0160278.

7. Simpson SQ. SIRS in the time of sepsis-3. Chest 2018;153(1):34–8.
8. Saeed K, Wilson DC, Bloos F, et al. The early identification of disease progression in patients with suspected infection presenting to the emergency department: a multicentre derivation and validation study. Crit Care 2019;23:40.
9. Kumar H, Kawai T, Akira S. Pathogen recognition by the innate immune system. Int Rev Immunol 2011;30(1):16–34.
10. Wiersinga WJ, Leopold SJ, Cranendonk DR, et al. Host innate immune response to sepsis. Virulence 2014;5(1):36–44.
11. Dolasia K, Bisht MK, Pradhan G, et al. TLRs/NLRs: shaping the landscape of host immunity. Int Rev Immunol 2018;37(1):3–19.
12. Faix JD. Biomarkers of sepsis. Crit Rev Clin Lab Sci 2013;50(1):23–36.
13. Bone RC, Balk RA, Cerra FB, et al. American College of Chest Physicians/Society of Critical Care Medicine Consensus Conference: definitions for sepsis and organ failure and guidelines for the use of innovative therapies in sepsis. Crit Care Med 1992;20(6):864–74.
14. Dellinger RP, Levy MM, Carlet JM, et al. Surviving sepsis campaign: international guidelines for management of severe sepsis and septic shock. Crit Care Med 2008;36:296–327.
15. Wunderink RG. Guidelines to manage community-acquired pneumonia. Clin Chest Med 2018;39:723–31.
16. Sungurlu S, Balk RA. The role of biomarkers in the diagnosis and management of pneumonia. Clin Chest Med 2018;39:691–701.
17. Ahnert P, Creutz P, Horn K, et al. Sequential organ failure assessment score is an excellent operationalization of disease severity of adult patients with hospitalized community-acquired pneumonia – results from the prospective observational PROGRESS study. Crit Care 2019;23(1):110.
18. Fernandez JF, Sibila O, Restrepo MI. Predicting ICU admission in community-acquired pneumonia: clinical scores and biomarkers. Expert Rev Clin Pharmacol 2012;5:445–58.
19. Zhydkov A, Christ-Crain M, Thomann R, et al. Utility of procalcitonin, C-reactive protein, and white blood cells alone and in combination for the prediction of clinical outcomes in community-acquired pneumonia. Clin Chem Lab Med 2015;53(4):559–66.
20. Seymour CW, Liu VX, Iwashyna TJ, et al. Assessment of clinical criteria for sepsis: for the third international consensus definitions for sepsis and septic shock (Sepsis-3). JAMA 2016;315(8):762–74.
21. Magadia RR, Weinstein MP. Laboratory diagnosis of bacteremia and fungemia. Infect Dis Clin North Am 2001;15:1009–24.
22. Riedel S, Carroll KC. Blood cultures: key elements for best practices and future directions. J Infect Chemother 2010;16:301–6.
23. Martin GS, Mannino DM, Eaton S, et al. The epidemiology of sepsis in the United States from 1979 through 2000. N Engl J Med 2003;348(16):1546–54.
24. Bochud PY, Bonten M, Marchetti O, et al. Antimicrobial therapy for patients with severe sepsis and septic shock: an evidence based review. Crit Care Med 2004;32(11 Suppl):S495–512.
25. Phua J, Ngerng WJ, See KC, et al. Characteristics and outcomes of culture-negative versus culture-positive severe sepsis. Crit Care 2013;17:R202.
26. Biomarkers Definitions Working Group, Bethesda MD. Biomarkers and surrogate endpoints: preferred definitions and conceptual framework. Clin Pharmacol Ther 2001;69:89–95.

27. Marshall JC, Reinhart K, International Sepsis Forum. Biomarkers of sepsis. Crit Care Med 2009;37(7):2290–8.

28. Pierrakos C, Vincent JL. Sepsis biomarker: a review. Crit Care 2010;14(1):R15.

29. Clinical Trials. List of open studies regarding "sepsis AND biomarkers" 2017. Available at: https://www.clinicaltrials.gov/ct2/results?term=sepsis+AND+biomarkers&rcr=open. Accessed April 9, 2019.

30. Clinical Trials. List of open studies regarding "pneumonia AND biomarkers" 2017. Available at: https://www.clinicaltrials.gov/ct2/results?term=pneumonia+AND+biomarkers&rcr=open. Accessed April 9, 2019.

31. Gluck E, Nguyen HB, Yalamanchili K, et al. Real-world use of procalcitonin and other biomarkers among sepsis hospitalizations in the United States: a retrospective, observational study. PLoS One 2018;13(10):e0205924.

32. Gabay C, Kushner I. Acute-phase proteins and other systemic responses to inflammation. N Engl J Med 1999;340:448–54.

33. Black S, Kushner I, Samols D. C-reactive protein. J Biol Chem 2004;279(47):48487–90.

34. Lelubre C, Anselin S, Zouaoui Boudjeltia K, et al. Interpretation of C-reactive protein concentrations in critically ill patients. Biomed Res Int 2013;2013:124021.

35. Vincent JL, Donadello K, Schmidt X. Biomarkers in the critically ill patient: C-reactive protein. Crit Care Clin 2011;27:241–51.

36. Eschborn S, Weitkamp JH. Procalcitonin versus C-reactive protein: review of kinetics and performance for diagnosis of neonatal sepsis. J Perinatol 2019. https://doi.org/10.1038/s41372-019-0363-4.

37. Riedel S, Carroll KC. Laboratory detection of sepsis: biomarkers and molecular approaches. Clin Lab Med 2013;33(3):413–37.

38. Nora D, Salluh J, Martin-Loeches I, et al. Biomarker-guided antibiotic therapy – strengths and limitations. Ann Transl Med 2017;5(10):208.

39. Mantovani A, Garlanda C, Doni A, et al. Pentraxins in innate immunity: from C-reactive protein to the long pentraxin PTX3. J Clin Immunol 2008;28:1–13.

40. Albert Vega C, Mommert M, Boccard M, et al. Source of circulating pentraxin 3 in septic shock patients. Front Immunol 2019;9:3048.

41. Inforzato A, Botazzi B, Garlanda C, et al. Pentraxins in humoral immunity. Adv Exp Med Biol 2012;946:1–20.

42. Mauri T, Bellani G, Patroniti N, et al. Persisting high levels of pentraxin 3 over the first days after severe sepsis and septic shock onset are associated with mortality. Intensive Care Med 2010;36:621–9.

43. Hamed S, Behnes M, Pauly D, et al. Diagnostic value of pentraxin-3 in patients with sepsis and septic shock in accordance with latest sepsis-3 definitions. BMC Infect Dis 2017;17(1):554.

44. deKruif MD, Limper M, Sierrhuis K, et al. PTX3 predicts severe disease in febrile patients in the emergency department. J Infect 2010;60:122–7.

45. Uusitalo-Seppälä R, Huttunen R, Aittoniemi J, et al. Pentraxin 3 (PTX3) is associated with severe sepsis and fatal disease in emergency room patients with suspected infection: a prospective cohort study. PLoS One 2013;8(1):e53661.

46. Riedel S. Procalcitonin and the role of biomarkers in the diagnosis and management of sepsis. Diagn Microbiol Infect Dis 2012;73:221–7.

47. Assicot M, Gendrel D, Carsin H, et al. High serum procalcitonin concentrations in patients with sepsis and infection. Lancet 1993;341:515–8.

48. Meisner M. Pathobiochemistry and clinical use of procalcitonin. Clin Chim Acta 2002;323(1–2):17–29.

49. Mueller B, White JC, Nylen ES, et al. Ubiquitous expression of the calcitonin-I gene in multiple tissues in response to sepsis. J Clin Endocrinol Metab 2001; 86:396–404.
50. Brunkhorst FM, Heinz U, Forycki ZF. Kinetics of procalcitonin in iatrogenic sepsis. Intensive Care Med 1998;24(8):888–9.
51. Becker KL, Nylen ES, White JC, et al. Procalcitonin and the calcitonin gene family of peptides in inflammation, infection, and sepsis: a journey from calcitonin back to its precursors. J Clin Endocrinol Metab 2004;89:1512–25.
52. Mueller B, Peri G, Doni A, et al. High circulating levels of the IL-1 type II decoy receptor in critically ill patients with sepsis: association of decoy receptor levels with glucocorticoid administration. J Leukoc Biol 2002;72:643–9.
53. Mueller B, Christ-Crain M, Bregenzer T, et al. Procalcitonin levels predict bacteremia in patients with community-acquired pneumonia: a prospective clinical trial. Chest 2010;138:121–9.
54. DeKruif M, Limper M, Gerritsen H, et al. Additional value of procalcitonin for diagnosis of infection in patients with fever in the emergency department. Crit Care Med 2010;38:457–63.
55. Riedel S, Meledez JH, An AT, et al. Procalcitonin as a marker for the detection of bacteremia and sepsis in the emergency department. Am J Clin Pathol 2011; 135:182–9.
56. Jeong S, Park Y, Cho Y, et al. Diagnostic utilities of procalcitonin and C-reactive protein for the prediction of bacteremia determined by blood culture. Clin Chim Acta 2012;413(21–22):1731–6.
57. Liu HH, Zhang MW, Guo JB, et al. Procalcitonin and C-reactive protein in early diagnosis of sepsis caused by either Gram-negative or Gram-positive bacteria. Ir J Med Sci 2017;186(1):207–12.
58. Thomas-Rüddel DO, Poidinger B, Kott M, et al. Influence of pathogen and focus of infection on procalcitonin levels in sepsis patients with bacteremia or candidemia. Crit Care 2018;22(1):128.
59. Schuetz P, Mueller B, Trampuz A. Serum procalcitonin for discrimination of blood contamination from bloodstream infection due to coagulase-negative staphylococci. Infection 2007;35:352–5.
60. Lai CC, Chen SY, Wang CY, et al. Diagnostic value of procalcitonin for bacterial infection in elderly patients in the emergency department. J Am Geriatr Soc 2010;58:518–22.
61. Fioretto JR, Martin JG, Kurokawa, et al. Comparison between procalcitonin and C-reactive protein for early diagnosis of children with sepsis and septic shock. Inflamm Res 2010;59:581–6.
62. Jones AE, Fiechtl JF, Brown MD, et al. Procalcitonin test in the diagnosis of bacteremia: a meta-analysis. Ann Emerg Med 2007;50:34–41.
63. Simon L, Gauvin F, Amre DK, et al. Serum procalcitonin and C-reactive protein levels as markers of bacterial infection: a systematic review and meta-analysis. Clin Infect Dis 2004;39:206–17.
64. Uzzan B, Cohen R, Nicolas P, et al. Procalcitonin as a diagnostic test for sepsis in critically ill adults after surgery or trauma: a systematic review and meta-analysis. Crit Care Med 2006;34:1996–2003.
65. Vouloumanou EK, Plessa E, Karageorgopoulos DE, et al. Serum procalcitonin as a diagnostic marker for neonatal sepsis: a systematic review and meta-analysis. Intensive Care Med 2011;37:747–62.

66. Wacker C, Prkno A, Brunkhorst FM, et al. Procalcitonin as a diagnostic marker for sepsis: a systematic review and meta-analysis. Lancet Infect Dis 2013; 14(5):426–35.

67. Pontrelli G, De Crescenzo F, Buzzetti R, et al. Accuracy of serum procalcitonin for the diagnosis of sepsis in neonates and children with systemic inflammatory syndrome: a meta-analysis. BMC Infect Dis 2017;17(1):302.

68. Kibe S, Adams K, Barlow G. Diagnostic and prognostic biomarkers of sepsis in critical care. J Antimicrob Chemother 2011;66(Suppl 2):33–40.

69. Ruiz-Alvarez MJ, Garcia-Valdecasas S, De Pablo R, et al. Diagnostic efficacy and prognostic value of serum procalcitonin concentration in patients with suspected sepsis. J Intensive Care Med 2009;24:63–71.

70. Nobre V, Harbarth S, Graf JD, et al. Use of procalcitonin to shorten antibiotic treatment duration in septic patients. Am J Respir Crit Care Med 2008;177: 498–505.

71. Bouadma L, Luyt CE, Tubach F, et al. Use of procalcitonin to reduce patients' exposure to antibiotics in intensive care units (PRORATA trial): a multicentre randomised controlled trial. Lancet 2010;375:463–74.

72. Agrawal R, Schwartz DN. Procalcitonin to guide duration of antimicrobial therapy in intensive care units: a systematic review. Clin Infect Dis 2011;53:379–87.

73. Schuetz P, Chiappa V, Briel M, et al. Procalcitonin algorithms for antibiotic therapy decisions: a systematic review of randomized controlled trials and recommendation for clinical algorithms. Arch Intern Med 2011;171:1322–31.

74. Schuetz P, Birkhahn R, Sherwin R, et al. Serial procalcitonin predicts mortality in severe sepsis patients: results from the Multicenter Procalcitonin Monitoring Sepsis (MOSES) study. Crit Care Med 2017;45(5):781–9.

75. Wirz Y, Meier MA, Bouadma L, et al. Effect of procalcitonin-guided antibiotic treatment on clinical outcomes in intensive care unit patients with infection and sepsis patients: a patient-level meta-analysis of randomized trials. Crit Care 2018;22:191.

76. Chu DC, Mehta AB, Walkey AJ. Practice patterns and outcomes associated with procalcitonin use in critically ill patients with sepsis. Clin Infect Dis 2017;64(11): 1509–15.

77. Hinson JP, Kapas S, Smith DM. Adrenomedullin, a multifunctional regulatory peptide. Endocr Rev 2000;21:138–67.

78. Hirata Y, Mitaka C, Sato K, et al. Increased circulating adrenomedullin, a novel vasodilatory peptide, in sepsis. J Clin Endocrinol Metab 1996;81:1449–53.

79. Christ-Crain M, Morgenthaler NG, Struck J, et al. Mid-regional proadrenomedullin as a prognostic marker in sepsis: an observational study. Crit Care 2005;9: R816–24.

80. Guignant C, Vorin N, Venet F, et al. Assessment of pro-vasopressin and pro-adrenomedullin as predictors of 28-day mortality in septic shock patients. Intensive Care Med 2009;35:1859–67.

81. Debiane L, Hachem RY, Al Wohoush I, et al. The utility of proadrenomedullin and procalcitonin in comparison to C-reactive protein as predictors of sepsis and bloodstream infection in critically ill patients with cancer. Crit Care Med 2014; 42(12):2500–7.

82. Gunnar E, Bloos F, Wilson DC, et al. The use of mid-regional proadrenomedullin to identify disease severity and treatment response to sepsis – a secondary analysis of a larger randomised controlled trial. Crit Care 2018;22:79.

83. Viaggi B, Poole D, Tujjar O, et al. Mid regional pro-adrenomedullin for the prediction of organ failure in infection. Results from a single centre study. PLoS One 2018;13(8):e0201491.

84. Analuz-Ojeda D, Nguyen HB, Meunier-Beillaerd N, et al. Superior accuracy of mid-regional proadrenomedullin for mortality prediction in sepsis with varying levels of illness severity. Ann Intensive Care 2017;7(1):15.

85. Li Q, Wang BS, Yang L, et al. Assessment of adrenomedullin and proadrenomedullin as predictors of mortality in septic patients: a systematic review and meta-analysis. Med Intensiva 2018;42(&):416–24.

86. Trzeciak S, Dellinger R, Chansky ME, et al. Serum lactate as a predictor of mortality in patients with infection. Intensive Care Med 2007;33:970–7.

87. Puskarich MA, Trzeciak S, Shapiro N, et al. Whole blood lactate kinetics in patients undergoing quantitative resuscitation for severe sepsis and septic shock. Chest 2013;143(6):1548–53.

88. Singer AJ, Taylor M, Domingo A, et al. Diagnostic characteristics of a clinical screening tool in combination with measuring bedside lactate level in emergency department patients with suspected sepsis. Acad Emerg Med 2014; 21(8):853–7.

89. Anderson LW, Mackenhauer J, Roberts JC, et al. Etiology and therapeutic approach to elevated lactate. Mayo Clin Proc 2013;88(10):1127–40.

90. Dugas AF, Mackenhauer J, Salciccioli JD, et al. Prevalence and characteristics of nonlactate and lactate expressors in septic shock. J Crit Care 2012;27(4): 344–50.

91. Kuster H, Weiss M, Willeitner AE, et al. Interleukin-1 receptor antagonist and interleukin-6 for early diagnosis of neonatal sepsis 2 days before clinical manifestations. Lancet 1998;352:1271–7.

92. Uusitalo-Seppälä R, Koskinen P, Leino A, et al. Early detection of severe sepsis in the emergency room: diagnostic value of C-reactive protein, procalcitonin, and interleukin-6. Scand J Infect Dis 2011;43:883–90.

93. Andaluz-Ojeda D, Bobillo F, Iglesias V, et al. A combined score of pro- and anti-inflammatory interleukins improves mortality prediction in severe sepsis. Cytokine 2012;57:332–6.

94. Meem M, Modak JK, Mortuza R, et al. Biomarkers for diagnosis of neonatal infections: a systematic analysis of their potential as a point-of-care diagnostics. J Glob Health 2011;1:201–9.

95. Bouchon A, Facchetii F, Weigand MA, et al. TREM-1 amplifies inflammation and is a crucial mediator of sepsis. Nature 2001;410:1103–7.

96. Wu Y, Wang F, Fan X, et al. Accuracy of plasma sTREM-1 for sepsis diagnosis in systemic inflammatory patients: a systematic review and meta-analysis. Crit Care 2012;16:R229.

97. Cao C, Gu J, Zhang J. Soluble triggering receptor expressed on myeloid cell-1 (sTREM-1): a potential biomarker for the diagnosis of infectious diseases. Front Med 2017;11:169–77.

98. Shozushima T, Takahashi G, Matsumoto M, et al. Usefulness of presepsin sCD14-ST measurements as a marker for the diagnosis and severity of sepsis that satisfied diagnostic criteria for systemic inflammatory response syndrome. J Infect Chemother 2011;17:764–9.

99. Endo S, Suzuki Y, Takahashi G, et al. Usefulness of presepsin in the diagnosis of sepsis in a multicenter prospective study. J Infect Chemother 2012;18:891–7.

100. Henriquez-Camacho C, Losa J. Biomarkers of sepsis. Biomed Res Int 2014; 2014:547818.

101. Christ-Crain M, Schuetz P, Mueller B. Biomarkers in the management of pneumonia. Expert Rev Respir Med 2008;2(5):565–72.
102. Mueller B, Harbarth S, Stolz D, et al. Diagnostic and prognostic accuracy of clinical and laboratory parameters in community-acquired pneumonia. BMC Infect Dis 2007;7:10.
103. Moulin F, Raymond J, Lorrot M, et al. Procalcitonin in children admitted to hospital with community acquired pneumonia. Arch Dis Child 2001;84(4):332–6.
104. Johansson N, Kalin M, Backman-Johansson C, et al. Procalcitonin levels in community-acquired pneumonia – correlation with aetiology and severity. Scand J Infect Dis 2014;46(11):787–91.
105. Suberviola B, Castellanos-Ortega A, Llorca J, et al. Prognostic value of proadrenomedullin in severe sepsis and septic shock with community-acquired pneumonia. Swiss Med Wkly 2012;142:w13542.
106. Cavallazzi R, El-Kersh K, Abu-Atherah E, et al. Midregional proadrenomedullin for prognosis in community-acquired pneumonia: a systematic review. Respir Med 2014;108(11):1569–80.
107. Schuetz P, Christ-Crain M, Thomann R, et al. Effect of procalcitonin-based guidelines vs. standard guidelines on antibiotic use in lower respiratory tract infections: the ProHOSP randomized controlled trial. JAMA 2009;302(10):1059–66.
108. Branche A, Neeser O, Mueller B, et al. Procalcitonin to guide antibiotic decision making. Curr Opin Infect Dis 2019;32(2):130–5.
109. Schuetz P, Wirz Y, Sager R, et al. Effect of procalcitonin-guided antibiotic treatment on mortality in acute respiratory infections: a patient-level meta-analysis. Lancet Infect Dis 2018;19(1):95–107.
110. Huang DT, Yealy DM, Filbin MR, et al. Procalcitonin-guided use of antibiotics for lower respiratory tract infection. N Engl J Med 2018;379(3):236–49.
111. Lam SW, Bauer SR, Fowler R, et al. Systematic review and meta-analysis of procalcitonin-guidance versus usual care for antimicrobial management in critically ill patients: focus on subgroups based on antibiotic initiation, cessation, or mixed strategies. Crit Care Med 2018;46:684–90.
112. Velissaris D, Pintea M, Pantzaris N, et al. The role of procalcitonin in the diagnosis of meningitis: a literature review. J Clin Med 2018;7(6):148.
113. Li W, Sun X, Yuan F, et al. Diagnostic accuracy of cerebrospinal fluid procalcitonin in bacterial meningitis patients with empiric antibiotic pretreatment. J Clin Microbiol 2017;55(4):1193–204.
114. Drozdov D, Schwartz S, Kutz A, et al. Procalcitonin and pyuria-based algorithm reduces antibiotic use in urinary tract infections: a randomized controlled trial. BMC Med 2015;13:104.
115. Serkova NJ, Standiford TJ, Stringer KA. The emerging field of quantitative blood metabolomics for biomarker discovery in critical illnesses. Am J Respir Crit Care 2011;184(6):647–55.
116. Goh C, Knight JC. Enhanced understanding of the host-pathogen interaction in sepsis: new opportunities for omic approaches. Lancet Respir Med 2017;5(3):212–23.
117. Sweeney TE, Wong HR, Khatri P. Robust classification of bacterial and viral infections via integrated host gene expression diagnostics. Sci Transl Med 2016;8(246):346ra91.
118. Vayssier-Taussat M, Albina E, Citti C, et al. Shifting the paradigm from pathogen to pathobiome: new concepts in the light of meta-omics. Front Cell Infect Microbiol 2014;4:29.

What the Clinical Microbiologist Should Know About Pharmacokinetics/ Pharmacodynamics in the Era of Emerging Multidrug Resistance
Focusing on β-Lactam/β-Lactamase Inhibitor Combinations

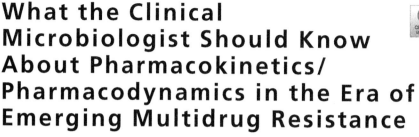

Henrietta Abodakpi, PharmD, PhD[a], Audrey Wanger, PhD[b],
Vincent H. Tam, PharmD[a,c],*

KEYWORDS

- Combination therapy • Pharmacokinetics/pharmacodynamics
- Susceptibility testing • Optimal dosing • Gram-negative bacteria

KEY POINTS

- The continued dissemination of β-lactamases among gram-negative bacteria presents a major challenge to the treatment of nosocomial infections.
- β-Lactamase inhibitors have been important in preserving the activity of β-lactam antibiotics against β-lactamase–producing gram-negative bacteria.
- At present, there are technical gaps in the development and evaluation of β-lactam/β-lactamase inhibitor combinations.
- Improved understanding of the joint action of these combinations will better inform dosing strategies and preserve their efficacy against evolving β-lactamase resistance.

Disclosures: V.H. Tam has received honorarium from Merck. The other authors have nothing to disclose.
Funding: V.H. Tam is supported by the National Institutes of Health (R01AI140287-01).
[a] Department of Pharmacological and Pharmaceutical Sciences, University of Houston College of Pharmacy, Houston, TX, USA; [b] Department of Pathology and Laboratory Medicine, McGovern Medical School, 6431 Fannin, Houston, Texas 77030, USA; [c] Department of Pharmacy Practice and Translational Research, University of Houston College of Pharmacy, 4849 Calhoun Road, Houston, TX 77204, USA
* Corresponding author. Department of Pharmacy Practice and Translational Research, University of Houston College of Pharmacy, 4849 Calhoun Road, Houston, TX 77204.
E-mail address: vtam@uh.edu

Clin Lab Med 39 (2019) 473–485
https://doi.org/10.1016/j.cll.2019.05.006
0272-2712/19/© 2019 Elsevier Inc. All rights reserved.

labmed.theclinics.com

INTRODUCTION

Antibiotic resistance poses one of the greatest medical threats to human health. According to the US Centers for Disease Control and Prevention (CDC), resistant bacteria account for more than 2 million illnesses and 23,000 deaths annually in the United States alone.[1] In health care settings, infections caused by resistant gram-negative bacteria may be especially challenging to treat because they often present with multiple mechanisms of resistance. These infections are commonly associated with inappropriate or suboptimal therapy. Several studies have shown that resistance in gram-negative bacteria leads to additional costs and length of hospitalization, as well as high morbidity and mortality.[2–7] Although resistance to key antibiotics continues to increase, there is a shortage of new drug candidates in early development for the treatment of gram-negative bacterial infections. Thus, there is a pressing need for a critical evaluation of how to optimally use existing agents and those under development.

Gram-negative bacteria are highly adaptable pathogens capable of intrinsic and acquired resistance to multiple classes of antibiotics. Resistance to these agents is mediated through a variety of mechanisms that include decreased permeability through loss of porins, extrusion of drug through overexpression of transmembrane efflux pumps, decreased binding of drugs through target mutations, and the production of inactivating enzymes (eg, β-lactamases or functional group transferases). Of these, the production of β-lactamases is one of the most commonly encountered resistance mechanisms.

Historically, the use of β-lactamase inhibitors in combination with β-lactams has been critical to circumventing β-lactamase–mediated resistance. However, conventional practices in the development and evaluation of these combinations may preclude optimal clinical use. This article highlights current practices of developing β-lactam/β-lactamase inhibitor combinations, and discusses avenues for improved testing/pairing of these combinations.

β-LACTAMASE–MEDIATED RESISTANCE

β-lactams are an important class of antibiotics used for the treatment of infections caused by gram-negative pathogens. They exert their activity by inhibiting penicillin-binding proteins required for bacterial cell wall synthesis. As a result of the widespread use of these β-lactams, β-lactamase–producing organisms have become a prominent concern.[8–12]

β-lactamases represent a heterogeneous group of enzymes capable of hydrolyzing and inactivating the core β-lactam ring required for the bactericidal activity of β-lactam antibiotics. These β-lactamases are classified either according to substrate and inhibitor profiles (Bush-Jacoby classification) or primary amino acid sequences (Ambler classification). The Ambler classification groups β-lactamases into classes A, B, C, and D, as shown in **Table 1**. In the United States, class A enzymes are the predominant β-lactamases reported in gram-negative species.[11–13] Genes encoding class A enzymes are generally located on plasmids that can be transferred between bacterial species. These enzymes include penicillinases, extended-spectrum β-lactamases (ESBLs), and carbapenemases. Penicillinases (eg, SHV-1, TEM-1) primarily hydrolyze penicillins and early-generation cephalosporins.[14,15] In addition to penicillins, ESBLs (eg, CTX-M and other SHV and TEM subtypes) hydrolyze nearly all cephalosporins and monobactams.[14] Class A carbapenemases (eg, *Klebsiella pneumoniae* carbapenemases [KPCs]) are especially daunting because they can confer resistance to all currently available β-lactams. Nonetheless, the prevalence of other non–class A β-lactamases is also increasing. Furthermore, many clinical isolates harbor multiple

Table 1
Major classes of β-lactamases of clinical importance

Ambler Class	Type of β-Lactamase	Preferred Substrates	Representative Enzymes
A	Narrow spectrum (penicillinase)	Penicillins, early cephalosporins	TEM-1/-2, SHV-1
A	Extended spectrum	Narrow-spectrum and extended-spectrum penicillins, cephalosporins	SHV-2, CTX-M-15
A	Serine carbapenemases	All β-lactams	KPC-2, KPC-3
B	Metallo-β-lactamases	β-lactams except aztreonam	IMP-1, VIM-1
C	Cephalosporinases	Cephalosporins	AmpC, CYM-2
D	Oxacillinases	Oxacillin/cloxacillin	OXA-1, OXA-2
D	Cephalosporinases	Oxacillin/cloxacillin, cephalosporins	OXA-11, OXA-15
D	Carbapenemases	Oxacillin, carbapenems	OXA-48

β-lactamase–encoding genes.[11,12] To circumvent these β-lactamases, several new β-lactamase inhibitors have been developed.

PHARMACOLOGY OF β-LACTAMASE INHIBITION

The use of β-lactamase inhibitors is considered one of the most successful approaches for restoring β-lactam efficacy and continues to be of interest in drug development. Currently approved β-lactamase inhibitors generally lack significant antibacterial effect at clinically relevant concentrations; instead, they inhibit β-lactamases to preserve the efficacy of partnering β-lactams. At present, they are unavailable commercially as standalone agents and are coformulated with a partner β-lactam. Existing combination products include piperacillin/tazobactam, ampicillin/sulbactam, amoxicillin/clavulanic acid, ceftazidime/avibactam, and meropenem/vaborbactam.

First-generation β-lactamase inhibitors (eg, sulbactam, clavulanic acid, and tazobactam) were designed structurally to resemble β-lactams. Their mechanism of inhibition involves irreversible binding to the β-lactamase active site to form an acyl-enzyme complex that is hydrolyzed into enzyme and inhibitor fragments.[16–18] Sulbactam, clavulanic acid, and tazobactam have in vitro inhibitory activity against class A penicillinases and extended-spectrum β-lactamases.[19] However, they lack inhibitory activity against class A (eg, KPC) and B carbapenemases (eg, NDM, IMP, and VIM), as well as class C (eg, AmpC) and D β-lactamases (eg, OXA enzymes; shown in **Table 1**).

Recently, avibactam and vaborbactam, which belong to distinct classes of non–β-lactam inhibitors, have been approved for clinical use. Avibactam and vaborbactam possess inhibitory activity against Ambler class A and C β-lactamases but lack activity against class B enzymes.[20,21] In addition, avibactam shows activity against selected class D enzymes.[20] These novel non–β-lactam inhibitors not only differ structurally from the traditional inhibitors; mechanistically, they bind reversibly to the enzyme active site without (in most cases) being hydrolyzed, which allows recycling of the inhibitor and potential binding to additional β-lactamase molecules.

Several other non–β-lactam inhibitors, such as relebactam, zidebactam, and nacubactam, are currently under clinical development. Relebactam is being designed for use with imipenem and has shown an inhibitory spectrum similar to that of avibactam.[21] Pharmacologically, zidebactam and nacubactam perform a unique hybrid function: inactivation of important β-lactamases (ie, KPCs, class D carbapenemases) as well as selective inhibition of penicillin-binding proteins, which may therefore also confer direct activity against metallo-β-lactamase–producing strains.[22,23] As a result of their unique mechanisms of action, these newer agents have the potential to address lingering challenges in the inhibition of clinically relevant β-lactamases.

EFFICACY OF β-LACTAM/β-LACTAMASE INHIBITOR COMBINATIONS

Although combinations such as piperacillin/tazobactam have been widely used for decades, in recent years there has been renewed interest in their utility against ESBL-producing Enterobacteriaceae. In the past, carbapenems have been considered the drug of choice for ESBL infections. However, the rapid dissemination of carbapenemases has highlighted the need to evaluate alternative treatment options. One of the first studies to explore the appropriateness of β-lactam/β-lactamase inhibitor combinations for ESBL bacteremia was a post hoc analysis featuring data from 6 prospective bacteremia cohorts. In that study, 30-day mortality and length of hospitalization for patients with ESBL Escherichia coli bacteremia were comparable for patients treated with β-lactam/β-lactamase inhibitor combinations (such as piperacillin/tazobactam) or a carbapenem.[24] Notably, the median piperacillin/tazobactam minimum inhibitory concentration (MIC) in that study was low (2/4 mg/L) given the current susceptibility breakpoint of less than or equal to 16/4 mg/L. In addition, the bacteremia cases were mostly caused by urinary and biliary infections, which are considered low to moderate inoculum infections. Following that landmark report, several observational clinical studies further evaluated the efficacy of piperacillin/tazobactam for ESBL bacteremia.

Although some studies have since validated these findings, there is a lack of consensus regarding the efficacy of piperacillin/tazobactam for ESBL infections. The outcomes of key studies are summarized in **Table 2**. Variables such as the pathogen involved, severity of infection (inoculum size), and primary infection site seem to affect the clinical efficacy of piperacillin/tazobactam.[24–29] These studies have generally suggested that piperacillin/tazobactam might be associated with positive outcomes for isolates presenting with low MICs (<8/4 mg/L), and for bacteremia secondary to low or moderate inoculum infections (such as urinary and biliary infections). Nonetheless, in a recent randomized clinical trial focusing on bloodstream infections caused by ESBL-producing E coli and K pneumoniae, treatment with piperacillin/tazobactam was associated with higher mortality than meropenem.[30] Consistent with the observational studies, lower mortalities (for the piperacillin/tazobactam treatment group) were observed in patients whose bacteremia was caused by urinary infections. The median piperacillin MICs were 2/4 mg/L for E coli isolates and 4/4 mg/L for K pneumoniae, whereas the overall median meropenem MIC was 0.023 mg/L. However, there did not seem to be a trend toward worsening outcomes at higher piperacillin/tazobactam MICs as noted in the observational studies. Taken altogether, the data from these studies highlight discrepancies between in vitro susceptibility and observed clinical efficacy for piperacillin/tazobactam.

Given the broader inhibitory spectra of the new inhibitors, combinations such as ceftazidime/avibactam and meropenem/vaborbactam have been evaluated primarily against carbapenemase-producing organisms. Although both combinations have shown efficacy against KPCs, there have already been reports of resistance to ceftazidime/avibactam. Clinical resistance was first reported for a K pneumoniae isolate harboring KPC-3 obtained from a patient who had no previous exposure to

Table 2
Studies comparing the efficacy of piperacillin/tazobactam versus carbapenems for extended-spectrum β-lactamase bacteremia

Investigator, Year	Study Design	Primary Organisms	Primary Infection Source	30-d Mortality			
				PTZ (%)	CBP (%)	P Value	Interpretation
Rodríguez-Baño,[24] 2012	Prospective	E coli	Urinary/biliary	9[a]	17	>.05	Comparable[b]
Harris et al,[25] 2015	Retrospective	E coli K pneumoniae	Urinary/biliary	8	17	>.05	Comparable
Tamma et al,[26] 2015	Retrospective	E coli K pneumoniae	Catheter	26	11	<.05	Inferior
Ofer-Friedman et al,[28] 2015	Retrospective	E coli K pneumoniae	Pneumonia	60	34	= .1[c]	Comparable[b]
Ng et al,[29] 2016	Retrospective	E coli K pneumoniae	Urinary	31	30	>.05	Comparable
Gutiérrez-Gutiérrez et al,[27] 2016	Retrospective	E coli K pneumoniae	Urinary	10	14	>.05	Comparable
Harris et al,[30] 2018	Prospective	E coli K pneumoniae	Urinary	12.3	3.7	= .90[d]	Inferior

Abbreviations: CBP, carbapenem; PTZ, piperacillin/tazobactam.
[a] Composite mortality associated with amoxicillin/clavulanic acid and piperacillin/tazobactam.
[b] Comparable within power of study to detect differences.
[c] P value shown for 30-day mortality; for 90-day mortality, $P<.05$.
[d] P value for noninferiority.

ceftazidime/avibactam.[31] Since that report, there have been clinical cases of resistance development following treatment with ceftazidime/avibactam in isolates harboring KPC-2 and KPC-3.[32,33] The rapid emergence of resistance soon after the commercial availability of ceftazidime/avibactam may further show shortcomings in the assessments and dosing of these combinations.

LIMITATIONS IN CURRENT PRACTICE WITH β-LACTAM/β-LACTAMASE INHIBITOR COMBINATIONS
Fixed Agent Pairings

The utility of β-lactams/β-lactamase inhibitors may be fundamentally limited by current practices in the design of these combinations. At present, β-lactams and β-lactamase inhibitors are paired most commonly based on shared pharmacokinetics (eg, similar elimination half-lives, biodistribution, and metabolic pathways). Although matching the pharmacokinetics of the 2 agents is key to ensuring the presence of both agents at the site of infection and protecting the integrity of the β-lactam antibiotic, these considerations alone may not ensure optimal efficacy against all clinical isolates. Furthermore, when more than 1 β-lactamase is present, individual enzymes may display different affinities and susceptibilities (to different β-lactamase inhibitors), thus a fixed agent combination may not always be optimal.

Fixed Dose Ratio Pairings

β-Lactam/β-lactamase inhibitor pairs are generally available only as a fixed dose ratio combination. For instance, commercial piperacillin/tazobactam formulations are all in 8:1 ratio (piperacillin to tazobactam). However, the rationale for this fixed ratio remains unclear. In some clinical scenarios (eg, enzyme hyperproduction or severe [high inoculum] infections) modification of this ratio may be necessary to ensure adequate inhibitor exposures. The exception to this practice is with oral formulations of amoxicillin/clavulanic acid, in which compositions of 2:1, 4:1, and 7:1 of β-lactam to β-lactamase inhibitor are available. These formulations allow some flexibility for clinicians to customize dosing to different clinical scenarios.

Current Approaches to Susceptibility Testing

Since the advent of β-lactamase inhibitors, there has been much debate regarding the most appropriate approach to assess in vitro susceptibility for β-lactam/β-lactamase inhibitor combinations. For some combinations, susceptibility is evaluated using a fixed inhibitor concentration (eg, 4 mg/L of tazobactam) with a range of concentrations for the β-lactam (reflective of dynamic concentrations observed in vivo). The resulting MIC is designated as susceptible, intermediate, or resistant based on established breakpoints for efficacy. This scheme is predicated on the assumption that the magnitude of enhanced susceptibility remains constant in the presence of an inhibitor, grossly neglecting the contribution that varying concentrations of inhibitor may have on susceptibility (**Fig. 1**).

Hence, only a partial assessment of efficacy may be achieved with a single inhibitor concentration, and the resulting susceptibility data may not always correlate with in vivo efficacy. For combinations such as ampicillin/sulbactam and amoxicillin/clavulanic acid, a fixed 2:1 ratio of β-lactam to inhibitor is used in susceptibility testing. For ampicillin/sulbactam, this approach reflects the 2:1 dose ratio used in all commercial formulations. Hence, it may be argued that this could better reflect the in vivo concentration ratio achieved for the combination and provide better insights into in vivo efficacy.[34,35] However, for amoxicillin/clavulanic acid, for which parenteral

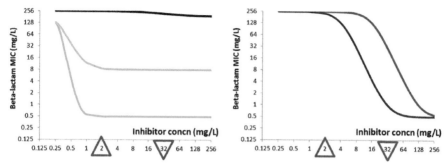

Fig. 1. Different hypothetical pharmacodynamic profiles of a β-lactamase inhibitor. A hypothetical β-lactamase inhibitor is known to have the following therapeutic concentration range with a standard dosing regimen: C_{max} = 32 mg/L (*inverted triangle*) and C_{min} = 2 mg/L (*upright triangle*). When used in combination with a β-lactam, various response profiles (ie, MIC reduction) can be anticipated for bacteria expressing different β-lactamases: black, minimal change in susceptibility (inactive inhibitor); green, dramatic reduction in susceptibility below C_{min}, minimal change over the therapeutic range (ideal active inhibitor); gold, moderate reduction in susceptibility below C_{min}, minimal change over the therapeutic range (active inhibitor rendered ineffective by other nonenzymatic resistance mechanisms); purple, gradual reduction in susceptibility over the therapeutic range (typical active inhibitor); pink, minimal change in susceptibility over the therapeutic range but gradual reduction above the therapeutic range (potentially active inhibitor with more aggressive dosing). concn, concentration.

formulations use a fixed ratio of 5:1 and oral formulations use varied dose ratios, the correlation between susceptibility testing ratios and anticipated in vivo ratios is less clear.

Conventional Pharmacokinetic/Pharmacodynamic Characterization of Combinations

Pharmacokinetic/pharmacodynamic (PK/PD) indices such as the maximum concentration divided by the MIC (C_{max}/MIC), the area under the 24-hour concentration-time curve divided by the MIC (AUC/MIC), and the percentage of free-time above MIC (%fT>MIC) are commonly used to characterize killing profiles for various antibiotics (**Fig. 2**). For β-lactams such as piperacillin and ceftazidime, the PK/PD index that best correlates with efficacy is the fT>MIC, which represents the duration of the dosing interval that the β-lactam concentration exceeds the MIC.

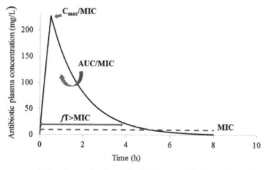

Fig. 2. PK/PD indices used to characterize the killing activity of various antibiotics. In all cases, the MIC (*red dashed line*) is expected to remain unchanged over time.

Understanding of the PK/PD of the β-lactam in combination with a β-lactamase inhibitor is more limited. When an inhibitor is coadministered, it is commonly assumed to have a fixed effect over the entire concentration range observed during a dosing interval (see **Fig. 1**). Although traditional inhibitors lack appreciable intrinsic killing, they are more likely to affect susceptibility in a concentration-dependent manner, as shown in **Fig. 1**. Thus, the assumption of a fixed (all or nothing) inhibitory effect may not always be appropriate and may hamper efforts to optimally dose these combinations.

ALTERNATIVE STRATEGIES FOR PAIRING AND ASSESSING β-LACTAM/β-LACTAMASE INHIBITOR COMBINATIONS

Evaluating the complex interplay between a β-lactam, β-lactamase inhibitor, and an infectious organism is not a trivial task. There is a critical need to address limitations in the current paradigm to guide rational pairing and dosing of β-lactam/β-lactamase inhibitor combinations. Several approaches have been proposed to improve the understanding of the dynamics of these combinations and to better inform dosing.

β-Lactamase Inhibitors as Standalone Agents

There are no standard regulatory pathways with respect to the development of β-lactamase inhibitors alone. The availability of standalone inhibitors would allow much-needed flexibility in these pairings to suit unique clinical needs. In addition, it would allow the tailoring of inhibitor doses to accommodate clinical isolates that express different degrees of enzyme activity. Experimental data suggest that a flexible pairing/dosing scheme could be instrumental to inhibiting isolates that do not respond to a conventional fixed ratio or fixed β-lactam/β-lactamase inhibitor pair.[36,37] In this scheme, pharmacokinetic considerations would remain relevant because dosing agents with dissimilar half-lives in tandem could be implemented by asymmetric dosing frequency (ie, dosing the 2 agents independently at different intervals) to reduce accumulation of the drug with the longer half-life. Furthermore, other approaches, such as staggered dosing (ie, dosing the β-lactam first and the β-lactamase inhibitor later after a lag time), could also maximize the effect of the agent combination in selected cases. Clinical microbiology testing could be used to guide selection of combinations and optimize ratios of the components.

Pharmacokinetic/Pharmacodynamic Index to Characterize the Effect of β-Lactamase Inhibitor

Using tazobactam as a reference inhibitor, Nicasio and colleagues[38] evaluated the PK/PD determinant that best predicts efficacy within the context of a fixed β-lactam (piperacillin) exposure. This study also evaluated the impact of β-lactamase gene transcription (low, moderate, and high) on the magnitude of PK/PD associated with efficacy. Using data from MIC studies, the percentage of time above a threshold inhibitor concentration (%Time>threshold) was identified as the index that best correlated to tazobactam efficacy. This threshold value signified a critical concentration (dependent on enzyme transcription levels) at which enzyme inhibition was maximal. These findings suggested that tazobactam exposures may need to be customized for individual isolates (based on differences in enzyme expression) to meet efficacy targets. From a dosing perspective, this approach is more informative than the current scheme, in which a fixed concentration of inhibitor (irrespective of β-lactamase activity) is used to show in vitro efficacy. However, it may still overlook inhibitor effects below and above the threshold concentration, and thus provides an incomplete overview of inhibitor pharmacodynamics.

Characterization of a Unique Pharmacokinetic/Pharmacodynamic Index Accounting for the Effect of Both the Inhibitor and the β-Lactam

To address similar issues, Bhagunde and colleagues[39] used relebactam (previously MK7655) in combination with imipenem against KPC-producing *K pneumoniae* to show the combined effects of a β-lactam and β-lactamase inhibitor. A full factorial design was used to explore susceptibility to the combination. MICs were determined using a range of inhibitor concentrations (as opposed to using a single fixed concentration) to better reflect the fluctuations in inhibitor concentration observed in vivo, and adapted to a modified inhibitory sigmoid E_{max} model (as shown in **Fig. 3**):

$$\log_2(MIC) = \log_2(MIC_0) - I_{max}I^H / \left(I^H + IC_{50}^H\right)$$

In this model, *MIC* is MIC in the presence of inhibitor; MIC_0 is MIC in the absence of inhibitor; I_{max} is maximum inhibitor effect; *H* is sigmoidicity coefficient; *I* is inhibitor concentration; and IC_{50} is inhibitor concentration required for 50% maximal inhibition. The model was used to characterize a theoretic concept known as the instantaneous MIC (MICi), which reflected changing pathogen susceptibility as inhibitor concentrations oscillated over a typical dosing interval. Bhagunde and colleagues[39] elaborated

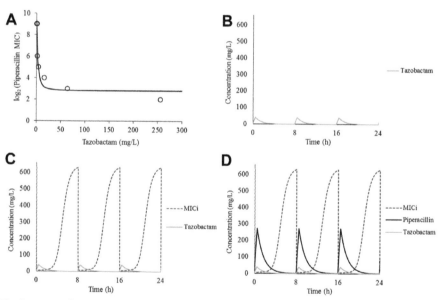

Fig. 3. MIC as function of inhibitor concentration and estimation of %*f*T>instantaneous MIC (MICi). Piperacillin MICs for a clinical isolate were determined in the presence of tazobactam concentrations ranging from 0 to 256 mg/L and modeled using the sigmoid inhibitory E_{max} model (*A*) to generate isolate-specific model parameter estimates. A free (unbound) tazobactam pharmacokinetic profile associated with a 0.5-g dose delivered every 8 hours was then simulated (*B*) and integrated with the E_{max} model parameter estimates to simulate a theoretic MICi profile (*C*). In contrast with the common approach, the MICi profile (*red dashed line*) reflected changing pathogen susceptibility as the inhibitor concentration fluctuated over time. In addition, a simulated unbound piperacillin pharmacokinetic profile associated with a 4-g dose every 8 hours was superimposed on the theoretic MICi profile (*D*). The %*f*T>MICi was then estimated as the duration of the dosing interval over which the piperacillin concentration exceeded the MICi (*f*T>MICi = 39.6% in *D*).

on this concept to define the percentage of free-time above instantaneous MIC (fT>MICi) as the PK/PD index that best correlated with the efficacy of imipenem/relebactam. Because MICi (a surrogate for susceptibility) depends on the relationship between individual β-lactamase–producing isolates and the inhibitor, this framework could be used to evaluate the efficacy of various β-lactamase inhibitor exposures against individual isolates. This approach is shown in **Fig. 3** using piperacillin/tazobactam and an ESBL-producing clinical K pneumoniae isolate. In a small collection of ESBL-producing isolates, exposures of piperacillin/tazobactam yielding fT>MICi greater than or equal to 55.1% were observed to suppress bacterial growth.[36] Although the model is simple, additional operational elements (such as automated computation) would be needed in clinical settings to generate the more robust susceptibility profiling data required for optimal dosing recommendations.

Future Application in the Clinical Microbiology Laboratory: Susceptibility Profiling Based on a Concentration Ratio (Truncated Factorial Design)

When a β-lactam and a β-lactamase inhibitor have very similar pharmacokinetics, the concentrations of the agents are expected to remain at a fixed proportion at the site of infection over a dosing interval. In this context, the concept of susceptibility profiling can be abbreviated to testing a fixed ratio of the agents, based on the dose ratio of the formulation administered. For example, meropenem/vaborbactam is administered clinically as a 1:1 ratio. A strategy for susceptibility testing is to use meropenem/vaborbactam in a similar ratio, such as 64/64 mg/L, 32/32 mg/L, 16/16 mg/L, 8/8 mg/L, and 4/4 mg/L. Extending the fixed ratio method to various β-lactam/β-lactamase inhibitor combinations would provide a simple, easily implemented approach for automated in vitro susceptibility testing that could better reflect PK/PD knowledge for these agents. This topic should be an area of increased investigation by organizations such as the Clinical And Laboratory Standards Institute that provide guidance on antimicrobial susceptibility testing constituents. If further evidence for strain-dependent threshold effects is obtained based on β-lactamase expression and inhibitor engagement, then testing of fixed critical breakpoint concentrations of β-lactam with different concentrations of inhibitor may also provide data for individualized dosing strategies against specific pathogens.

WHAT RESEARCH IS NEEDED IN THE FUTURE?

In clinical settings, the ideal method for evaluating these combinations would have to provide informative insights and a quick turnaround time for bedside decisions to be made. In the long run, increasing involvement of robotics and artificial intelligence in automated platforms seems inevitable. Moreover, innovations in microfluidic design and liquid handling could promote the development of point-of-care devices to expedite identification and antimicrobial susceptibility profiling.

In the foreseeable future (next 5–10 years), advancements in whole-genome sequencing could lead the way forward by facilitating timely identification of enzyme-encoding genes in clinical isolates. This work could be leveraged to rule out β-lactamase inhibitor pairings (eg, selection of avibactam in the presence of metallo-β-lactamases). However, detection of β-lactamase genes alone lends no additional information on the degree of functional gene expression, thus potentially limiting the ability to individualize therapy. Given the potential differences in β-lactamase present, levels of gene expression, and substrate affinity among different clinical isolates, customizable β-lactam/β-lactamase inhibitor regimens could ensure the appropriate selection and dosing of inhibitors. Allowing some flexibility in the selection and dose of inhibitor could also improve clinical efficacy and/or delay the development of resistance against these combinations. Nonetheless, regulatory hurdles and concerns about medication errors could hinder the commercialization of standalone inhibitors. With the continued discovery of more sophisticated inhibitors, improved methods for the in vitro evaluation of β-lactam/β-lactamase inhibitor combinations in the clinical microbiology laboratory are warranted.

SUMMARY

The continued dissemination of multidrug-resistant bacteria is an inevitable consequence of antibiotic use. β-Lactam/β-lactamase inhibitor combinations remain viable options for the treatment of infections caused by β-lactamase–producing bacteria and could help address worsening resistance. However, current susceptibility testing practices do not provide the best guidance for β-lactam/β-lactamase inhibitor therapy. New approaches based on evolving understanding of PK/PD for combination therapy are needed to guide clinicians in the optimal selection and rational dosing of these combinations.

REFERENCES

1. Centers for Disease Control and Prevention. Antibiotic resistance threats in the United States, 2013. 2014. Available at: https://www.cdc.gov/drugresistance/threat-report-2013/index.html. Accessed October 24, 2018.
2. Slama TG. Gram-negative antibiotic resistance: there is a price to pay. Crit Care 2008;12(Suppl 4):S4.
3. Cerceo E, Deitelzweig SB, Sherman BM, et al. Multidrug-resistant gram-negative bacterial infections in the hospital setting: overview, implications for clinical practice, and emerging treatment options. Microb Drug Resist 2016;22(5):412–31.
4. Tam VH, Rogers CA, Chang K-T, et al. Impact of multidrug-resistant pseudomonas aeruginosa bacteremia on patient outcomes. Antimicrob Agents Chemother 2010;54(9):3717–22.
5. Mauldin PD, Salgado CD, Hansen IS, et al. Attributable hospital cost and length of stay associated with health care-associated infections caused by antibiotic-resistant gram-negative bacteria. Antimicrob Agents Chemother 2010;54(1):109–15.
6. Ibrahim EH, Sherman G, Ward S, et al. The influence of inadequate antimicrobial treatment of bloodstream infections on patient outcomes in the ICU setting. Chest 2000;118(1):146–55.
7. Kollef MH, Sherman G, Ward S, et al. Inadequate antimicrobial treatment of infections: a risk factor for hospital mortality among critically ill patients. Chest 1999;115(2):462–74.
8. Adler A, Katz DE, Marchaim D. The continuing plague of extended-spectrum beta-lactamase-producing enterobacteriaceae infections. Infect Dis Clin North Am 2016;30(2):347–75.
9. Paterson DL. Resistance in gram-negative bacteria: enterobacteriaceae. Am J Med 2006;119(6 Suppl 1):S20–8 [discussion: S62–70].
10. Ruppe E, Woerther PL, Barbier F. Mechanisms of antimicrobial resistance in gram-negative bacilli. Ann Intensive Care 2015;5(1):61.
11. Castanheira M, Farrell SE, Deshpande LM, et al. Prevalence of β-lactamase-encoding genes among Enterobacteriaceae bacteremia isolates collected in 26 U.S. hospitals: report from the SENTRY antimicrobial surveillance program (2010). Antimicrob Agents Chemother 2013;57(7):3012–20.

12. Castanheira M, Farrell SE, Krause KM, et al. Contemporary diversity of β-lacta-mases among enterobacteriaceae in the nine U.S. Census regions and ceftazidime-avibactam activity tested against isolates producing the most preva-lent β-lactamase groups. Antimicrob Agents Chemother 2014;58(2):833–8.
13. Nordmann P, Naas T, Poirel L. Global spread of carbapenemase-producing enterobacteriaceae. Emerg Infect Dis 2011;17(10):1791–8.
14. Bush K. Bench-to-bedside review: the role of β-lactamases in antibiotic-resistant gram-negative infections. Crit Care 2010;14(3):224.
15. Bush K, Jacoby GA. Updated functional classification of β-lactamases. Antimi-crob Agents Chemother 2010;54(3):969–76.
16. Bush K. Beta-lactamase inhibitors from laboratory to clinic. Clin Microbiol Rev 1988;1(1):109–23.
17. Wright AJ. The penicillins. Mayo Clin Proc 1999;74(3):290–307.
18. Drawz SM, Bonomo RA. Three decades of beta-lactamase inhibitors. Clin Micro-biol Rev 2010;23(1):160–201.
19. Bush K. A resurgence of beta-lactamase inhibitor combinations effective against multidrug-resistant Gram-negative pathogens. Int J Antimicrob Agents 2015; 46(5):483–93.
20. Drawz SM, Papp-Wallace KM, Bonomo RA. New beta-lactamase inhibitors: a therapeutic renaissance in an MDR world. Antimicrob Agents Chemother 2014; 58(4):1835–46.
21. Wong D, van Duin D. Novel beta-lactamase inhibitors: unlocking their potential in therapy. Drugs 2017;77(6):615–28.
22. Sader HS, Castanheira M, Huband M, et al. WCK 5222 (Cefepime-Zidebactam) antimicrobial activity against clinical isolates of gram-negative bacteria collected worldwide in 2015. Antimicrob Agents Chemother 2017;61(5) [pii:e00072-17].
23. Moya B, Barcelo IM, Bhagwat S, et al. Potent β-lactam enhancer activity of zidebac-tam and WCK 5153 against Acinetobacter baumannii, including carbapenemase-producing clinical isolates. Antimicrob Agents Chemother 2017;61(11) [pii: e01238-17].
24. Rodriguez-Bano J, Navarro MD, Retamar P, et al, Beta-Lactamases–Red Espa-ñola de Investigación en Patología Infecciosa/Grupo de Estudio de Infección Hospitalaria Group. β-Lactam/β-lactam inhibitor combinations for the treatment of bacteremia due to extended-spectrum β-lactamase-producing Escherichia coli: a post hoc analysis of prospective cohorts. Clin Infect Dis 2012;54(2): 167–74.
25. Harris PN, Yin M, Jureen R, et al. Comparable outcomes for beta-lactam/beta-lactamase inhibitor combinations and carbapenems in definitive treatment of bloodstream infections caused by cefotaxime-resistant Escherichia coli or Kleb-siella pneumoniae. Antimicrob Resist Infect Control 2015;4:14.
26. Tamma PD, Han JH, Rock C, et al. Carbapenem therapy is associated with improved survival compared with piperacillin-tazobactam for patients with extended-spectrum beta-lactamase bacteremia. Clin Infect Dis 2015;60(9): 1319–25.
27. Gutiérrez-Gutiérrez B, Perez-Galera S, Salamanca E, et al. A multinational, pre-registered cohort study of beta-lactam/beta-lactamase inhibitor combinations for treatment of bloodstream infections due to extended-spectrum-beta-lactamase-producing enterobacteriaceae. Antimicrob Agents Chemother 2016; 60(7):4159–69.
28. Ofer-Friedman H, Shefler C, Sharma S, et al. Carbapenems versus piperacillin-tazobactam for bloodstream infections of nonurinary source caused by

extended-spectrum beta-lactamase-producing enterobacteriaceae. Infect Control Hosp Epidemiol 2015;36(8):981–5.
29. Ng TM, Khong WX, Harris PNA, et al. Empiric piperacillin-tazobactam versus carbapenems in the treatment of bacteraemia due to extended-spectrum beta-lactamase-producing enterobacteriaceae. PLoS One 2016;11(4):e0153696.
30. Harris PNA, Tambyah PA, Lye DC, et al. Effect of piperacillin-tazobactam vs meropenem on 30-day mortality for patients with E coli or Klebsiella pneumoniae bloodstream infection and ceftriaxone resistance: a randomized clinical trial. JAMA 2018;320(10):984–94.
31. Humphries RM, Yang S, Hemarajata P, et al. First report of ceftazidime-avibactam resistance in a KPC-3-expressing Klebsiella pneumoniae isolate. Antimicrob Agents Chemother 2015;59(10):6605–7.
32. Shields RK, Chen L, Cheng S, et al. Emergence of ceftazidime-avibactam resistance due to Plasmid-Borne bla$_{KPC-3}$ mutations during treatment of carbapenem-resistant Klebsiella pneumoniae infections. Antimicrob Agents Chemother 2017; 61(3) [pii:e02097-16].
33. Giddins MJ, Macesic N, Annavajhala MK, et al. Successive emergence of ceftazidime-avibactam resistance through distinct genomic adaptations in bla$_{KPC-2}$-harboring Klebsiella pneumoniae sequence type 307 isolates. Antimicrob Agents Chemother 2018;62(3) [pii:e02101-17].
34. Thomson CJ, Miles RS, Amyes SG. Susceptibility testing with clavulanic acid: fixed concentration versus fixed ratio. Antimicrob Agents Chemother 1995; 39(11):2591–2.
35. Pfaller MA, Barry AL, Fuchs PC, et al. Comparison of fixed concentration and fixed ratio options for dilution susceptibility testing of gram-negative bacilli to ampicillin and ampicillin/sulbactam. Eur J Clin Microbiol Infect Dis 1993;12(5): 356–62.
36. Abodakpi H, Chang K-T, Gao S, et al. Optimal piperacillin-tazobactam dosing strategies against extended-spectrum-β-lactamase-producing enterobacteriaceae. Antimicrob Agents Chemother 2019;63(2) [pii:e01906-18].
37. Abodakpi H, Chang KT, Zhou J, et al. A novel framework to compare the effectiveness of beta-lactamase inhibitors against extended-spectrum beta-lactamase-producing Enterobacteriaceae. Clin Microbiol Infect 2019. [Epub ahead of print].
38. Nicasio AM, VanScoy BD, Mendes RE, et al. Pharmacokinetics-pharmacodynamics of tazobactam in combination with piperacillin in an in vitro infection model. Antimicrob Agents Chemother 2016;60(4):2075–80.
39. Bhagunde P, Chang KT, Hirsch EB, et al. Novel modeling framework to guide design of optimal dosing strategies for beta-lactamase inhibitors. Antimicrob Agents Chemother 2012;56(5):2237–40.

Mapping the Road to the Future

Training the Next Generation of Clinical Microbiologists, from Technologist to Laboratory Director

Peter H. Gilligan, PhD, D(ABMM)[a],*, Martha H. McGee, BS, MT(ASCP)[b]

KEYWORDS

- Technologic change • Competencies • Medical laboratory scientists
- Training programs • Certification • Life-long learning • Clinical microbiology

KEY POINTS

- Rapid technologic change has transformed the very nature of the clinical microbiology discipline, making adaptability and life-long learning key professional competencies.
- Deemphasis of basic sciences, including microbiology in medical schools' curricula, requires greater levels of expertise among clinical microbiologists at all levels.
- New approaches to continuing medical education modeled on TED talks and YouTube videos should be developed by professional societies to appeal to the new generation of clinical microbiologists.
- The graying of the medical laboratory scientist workforce means greater opportunities at all staff levels in the clinical microbiology laboratory.
- Clinical microbiology laboratories may need to take creative approaches, such as apprenticeship-type programs, to fill an anticipated increasing number of vacancies.

INTRODUCTION

When one of the authors (P.H.G.) first started working in a clinical microbiology laboratory in the late 1970s, the available technology would have been very familiar to Pasteur: broth cultures, incubators, burners, and inoculating loops. However, even in the late 1970s, technology was in development that would automate the clinical microbiology laboratory beginning with the Bactec 460 used initially to detect microorganisms in blood cultures.[1,2] Over the next decade and a half, with the development of the

Disclosure Statement: The authors have nothing to disclose.
a Clinical Microbiology-Immunology Laboratories, UNC HealthCare, Chapel Hill, NC 27514, USA; b McLendon Clinical Laboratories, UNC HealthCare, Chapel Hill, NC 27514, USA
* Corresponding author.
E-mail address: celtsfan@med.unc.edu

Clin Lab Med 39 (2019) 487–497
https://doi.org/10.1016/j.cll.2019.05.007
0272-2712/19/© 2019 Elsevier Inc. All rights reserved.

labmed.theclinics.com

MicroScan and the Vitek systems, automation would allow the comparatively rapid identification and susceptibility of bacteria.[3] Soon after, the colorimetric detection of CO_2 resulting from microbial metabolism was applied to the automation of mycobacterial cultures and broth blood cultures.[4] The application of monoclonal antibodies to the rapid detection of microbial antigens directly in a variety of clinical specimens allowed real-time detection of several important human pathogens, including group A streptococci, *Cryptococcus neoformans*, *Clostridioides difficile*, *Legionella pneumophila*, *Chlamydia trachomatis*, respiratory syncytial virus (RSV), influenza virus, rotavirus, *Entamoeba histolytica*, *Giardia lamblia*, and *Cryptosporidium parvum*.[5]

The event that truly revolutionized diagnostic microbiology was the development of nucleic acid amplification technology (NAAT). The most widely used NAAT is the polymerase chain reaction (PCR), first extensively used in the 1990s.[6] A key diagnostic development in PCR technology was real-time PCR, which allows the rapid, sensitive, and specific detection of a wide array of microbial pathogens.[7] In particular, it has revolutionized clinical virology, replacing viral culture and antigen detection, and allowing important pathogens, such as RSV and influenza virus, to be detected during an office or emergency department visit.[8]

Multiplex NAAT tests have been successfully deployed for syndromic testing for the detection of organisms in blood cultures, feces, and respiratory secretions.[9] Its use in cerebrospinal fluid to detect agents of encephalitis and meningitis has been controversial and not as widely adopted.[10]

The combination of NAAT and sequencing technology has led to the 4 following important advances in microbial genomics:

1. Ribosomal sequencing for species identification of both bacteria and fungi;
2. Metagenomics analysis for pathogen discovery by using next-generation sequencing[11];
3. Whole-genome sequencing, which is now widely used for molecular epidemiology studies[12] with great promise for future applications; and
4. Microbiome analysis, which has greatly enhanced the understanding of chronic lung infection in cystic fibrosis and has been used to validate the therapeutic value of fecal microbial transplants.[13,14]

Proteomics is being applied to the identification of both bacteria and fungi. Matrix-assisted laser desorption/ionization–time-of-flight mass spectroscopy (MALDI-TOF MS) allows rapid identification of bacterial and fungal colonies in minutes to an hour depending on the level of preparation that is required before analysis.[15] Besides being rapid, it is easy to perform and inexpensive even when considering the capital expense.[16] This technology has replaced most other methods for identifying these organisms from culture in laboratories that can afford the capital investment.

Finally, robotics in the form of total laboratory automation (TLA) are becoming more common in larger laboratories that can afford the multi-million-dollar investment required to purchase and maintain the equipment. The promise of automation in the removal of repetitive, low-skill activities to free technologists for higher complexity tasks is appealing especially in a time when shortages of technologists due to a wave of retirements is becoming a reality.[17] Although outcome studies are currently limited, the combination of TLA and MALDI-TOF MS decreases time to reporting negative cultures, organism identifications, and antimicrobial susceptibility.[18–21] What is less certain is whether these decreased turnaround times translate into improved patient outcomes to justify this significant capital investment. The use of Artificial Intelligence for the reporting of negative cultures in TLA systems will further enhance efficiency, but again, will it improve outcomes?[22]

WHAT COMPETENCIES WILL BE NEEDED IN THE TWENTY-FIRST CENTURY MICROBIOLOGIST?

Clinical microbiologists at all levels will need specific competencies. Two interdependent competencies will be needed at all levels. First, all clinical microbiologists will need to be *life-long learners*. Pathogen discovery is ever increasing, driven by improved technology, urbanization, deforestation, antimicrobial pressure, industrial farming, climate change, and new therapies and organ transplants that extend the lives of immunologically vulnerable populations.[23] In order to be an effective life-long learner, all clinical microbiologists must be able to manage ever-increasing amounts of information.[23] Because the next clinical microbiology generation is "wired" as never before and obtains huge amounts of information visually, new approaches to gain this information in such venues as YouTube and TED Talks and the nascent video offerings of the Centers for Disease Control and Prevention (CDC) and respected journals, such as the *New England Journal of Medicine*, will need to be increased. Professional scientific societies, such as American Society for Microbiology, College of the American Pathologists, American Society for Clinical Pathologists, and Association of Molecular Pathologists, to name just a few, should increase their offerings of new information in easily digested formats similar to those found in TED Talks and YouTube.

With changes in medical education deemphasizing basic science knowledge,[24] clinicians have a more limited knowledge of microbiology at a time of ever-increasing complexity. In order to understand this increasingly complex world, microbiologists at all levels need good *analytical skills* so that they can assess the reliability of the information found electronically.

The days of a clinical microbiologist doing something because a clinician "says so" rather than doing what is microbiologically appropriate should be over because the clinical microbiologist is now, more than ever, the subject matter expert. Clinical microbiologists must have *superior communication and perhaps diplomatic skills*. In particular, clinical microbiologists at all levels, bench, supervisor/manager, and directors, should recognize the limits of their knowledge and work with related subject matter experts, especially infectious disease clinicians, pharmacists, and infection preventionists, to solve challenging clinical problems.

In order to do this effectively, the clinical microbiologist must be a *"good teammate,"* meaning sometimes doing things that might not make sense to them scientifically. The authors sometimes put such activities into the category of "treating the physician." The authors believe that treating physician colleagues well allows them to treat their patients well.

At all levels, *adaptability* is essential to success. The need for adaptability is driven by the rapid change in technologies. TLA, for example, requires reading culture plates on a computer screen rather than in one's hands. The sniffing of plates, perhaps never a wise practice but one, nevertheless, widely used, is not practical in a TLA setting. Simple biochemical tests, such as oxidase and catalase, are infrequently used. The rapid identification of microbes using conventional tests has given way to MALDI-TOF MS and chromogenic agars.[15,25]

Finally, all levels of microbiologists must have *superior computer skills*. Clinical microbiologists have used laboratory information systems for at least 3 decades. However, the widespread use of the electronic medical record (EMR) has created new challenges for the microbiologist. The authors have one of the most widely used EMRs, EPIC, and its laboratory information system companion, BEAKER, in their health care system. As one of their supervisors said, "There are many ways to order a test in EPIC, but only one way is correct." Over the past 3 years of using EPIC, count-less hours have been spent in trying to improve the ability to identify the specimen type correctly and report results that communicate what the authors found in a manner that is understood by the care provider. At face value, this appears fairly straightforward but has proven much more complex in reality. Because laboratory test–associated medical errors are most likely to occur at either the preanalytical or postanalytical stage,[26] assuring that computer issues are not the source of these errors is critical.

At the manager and doctoral level, writing skills are essential for development of easy-to-follow procedures that clearly explain how to use increasingly complex tech-nologies and communications to the care providers that are both succinct and easily understood. In both forms of communication, jargon and difficult-to-understand ab-breviations should be avoided.

At the doctoral level, clinical microbiologists are the true "experts." As such, one of the most important competencies one should have is to *know the limits of one's knowl-edge* or, put simply, being able to say, *"I don't know."* In particular, the doctoral-level scientists should be familiar with the key principles of clinical practice guidelines as they relate to their area of expertise. A working knowledge of infectious disease/clin-ical microbiology guidelines published by Clinical Laboratory Science Institute, Amer-ican Society for Microbiology, and Infectious Disease Society of America is essential. Doctoral scientists who are American Society for Microbiology members can access the ClinMicroNet. ClinMicroNet is a listserv with close to 900 members globally who discuss clinical problems in real time. It is an invaluable practice resource.

In institutions that do not have board-certified microbiologists, the clinical microbi-ology laboratory managers/supervisors must develop networks that allow them to be able to ask questions of trusted sources. Developing a trusted in-house network of cli-nicians, pharmacists, nurse managers, and infection preventionists is essential. Refer-ence laboratories that offer technical advice can be very helpful. Laboratories in "feeder hospitals" for large health care systems should rely on the experts at their reference institution. In addition, the American Society for Microbiology provides a list-serv for nondoctoral scientists that can play a similar role to the ClinMicroNet.

With the rapid expansion of genomic and proteomic knowledge, the doctoral-level scientist must be able to *use clinical applications based on this knowledge.* Doctoral-level scientists must have a working knowledge of biostatistics, molecular genomics as it relates to whole-genome and next-generation sequencing and microbiome anal-ysis, and the principles of mass spectroscopy.

Because of the significant capital expense necessary for the twenty-first century clinical microbiology laboratory, the managers and doctoral scientists need to be able to *manage up.* To effectively do this, they have to understand basic financial prin-ciples and develop strategic planning skills. They should be familiar with the basics of calculating a return on investment index and how to prepare a business plan. These skills are essential for communicating with hospital administration on financial pro-posals. In other words, they need to speak a hospital administrator's language so they can make the argument justifying large capital expenditure in this era of labora-tory automation. The argument is best made by showing clinical effectiveness, such as reduced patient stays as inpatient, and in the emergency department, and increased laboratory efficiencies that yield decreased costs.

Two other important competencies are *being a good teammate* and *mentoring.* The Centers of Medicare and Medicaid Services' emphasis on reduction of health care–associated conditions has resulted in the authors' institution forming several multidis-ciplinary teams to address infectious disease problems, such as *C difficile* infections, catheter-related urinary tract infections, and catheter-related bloodstream infections.[27] Clinical microbiologists serve on all of those teams in the authors' institution. In those setting, the microbiologist needs to be a "good teammate" in solving these problems even though they may have to compromise on certain aspects of the planned intervention. The Joint Commission requires all health care institutions to have an antimicrobial stewardship team with clinical microbiologists playing an essential role on that team.

Finally, doctoral-level clinical microbiologists, especially in teaching institutions, should endeavor to be effective mentors for undergraduate and graduate students, including medical students, pathology residents, and infectious disease and medical microbiology fellows. Mentoring takes both time and commitment to the mentee. However, the rewards are great for the mentee and for the discipline. Given the time pressures inherent in directing a complex organization, mentoring may have little appeal. However, it is important to remember how we got to where we are.

CHALLENGES IN TRAINING THE TWENTY-FIRST CENTURY CLINICAL MICROBIOLOGISTS

A recent survey showed a national vacancy rate of 6% for clinical microbiologists.[17] However, the situation may prove to be direr than that. TLA and rapid molecular testing are clinically most effective if the laboratory is staffed with medical laboratory scientists (MLSs) and medical laboratory technicians (MLTs) during evening and overnight shifts, shifts that have become increasingly difficult to staff. Without appropriate human resources, these technologic efficiencies may be lost.

Perhaps even more concerning is an estimated 25% of public health workers, including laboratorians, are planning to retire in the next 2 years.[28] Staffing shortages in public health laboratories may exacerbate the ability to respond to public health emergencies, such as tracking the epidemiology of food-borne illnesses, sexually transmitted infections, especially extremely drug-resistant gonococci, and other multidrug-resistant organisms, such as carbapenem-resistant Enterobacteriaceae.

According to a position paper of the American Society for Clinical Laboratory Science, the following 4 factors may drive increased vacancy rates among bench and supervisory technologists[29]:

1. Retirement among an aging workforce
2. An increased demand for testing driven in part by improved health care access due to the Affordable Care Act
3. Changes in practice due to increased test complexity and point-of-care testing oversight
4. Graduation rates from MLS and MLT programs that are not sufficiently high to meet increased workforce demands

Further complicating this issue are data that show a decreasing number of MLS and MLT programs and significant retirements among faculty of those programs especially among individuals in leadership positions.[29] What impact the retirement of faculty will have on the quality and quantity of programs is not clear. For programs that do exist, especially online ones, finding practicum sites is becoming increasingly difficult as workload demands reduce the willingness of clinical sites to take additional students or in some instances any students at all.[29]

The problem is further complicated by the fact that the Department of Labor Statistics estimated an approximately 20% growth rate in both MLS and MLT jobs.[30] Although the number of new clinical microbiology positions are not clear, they will likely increase as well.

A potential solution is for larger laboratories to develop laboratory training/apprentice programs for college graduates with science degrees that will prepare them through an alternate pathway for specialty certification examination in microbiology offered by the American Society of Clinical Pathology (ASCP). University of California, Los Angeles (UCLA) has a developed a 1-year Clinical Microbiology Scientist Program that is offered to individuals who have graduated with an undergraduate degree in microbiology and meets the ASCP educational requirements, which will allow participants to sit for the ASCP microbiology specialty certification examination.[23]

Retirement among clinical microbiology laboratory supervisors and managers will likely result in higher vacancy rates.[17,30] In the authors' experience, few technologists come to them expressing an interest in becoming a laboratory manager. Perhaps this is because there is no clear career ladder to become a laboratory manager at most institutions. Although there are numerous courses including online courses for Master of Business Administration, Master Degree in Management, and Master Degree in Health Care Administration, there are only a few Masters in Clinical Laboratory Management (examples include Rush University in Chicago and Michigan State University). Individuals who advance to become managers in most settings choose a route by becoming engaged in quality improvement or other managerial projects within the laboratory first and then pursuing Master level degrees when it becomes apparent that this is a promising career path for them.

At the doctoral level, there has been a wave of retirements, although data on vacancy rates are not available. Anecdotally though, recruitment of doctoral-level clinical microbiologist has been challenging especially in the public health laboratory setting. For staff appointments in many health care systems or to serve as the director of a high complexity laboratory as defined by Clinical Laboratory Improvement Amendments (CLIA), board certification as a medical microbiologist is required. There are 3 pathways that are widely used to fulfill this requirement. Two of the pathways begin with an earned doctoral degree followed by a fellowship in medical microbiology. These fellowships have a required curriculum approved by the specific certifying board that must be completed before taking the certification examination. Accreditation Council for Graduate Medical Education (ACGME) programs in medical microbiology are 1-year fellowships that are only open to individuals with medical degrees. There currently are 15 accredited programs in the United States, although not all programs may have a fellow each year due in part to a lack of interest among pathology residents in careers in clinical pathology in large part because they are less lucrative or do not meet the professional interests of the individual. Another group of physicians who fill these positions is infectious disease fellows, whose professional interests are closely aligned with clinical microbiology. However, historically, only a relatively small number of these clinicians have chosen this route. With declining interest in infectious disease fellowships in the United States,[31] it is unlikely that this group will fill the gap of those medical microbiology fellowship positions. Individuals completing this fellowship are eligible to take the American Board of Pathology subspecialty certification examination in medical microbiology.

The American Society for Microbiology accredits 18 two-year medical microbiology programs through its Committee on Postdoctoral Educational Programs or CPEP. Individuals with an earned doctoral degree in the life sciences, public health, veterinary medicine, dentistry, or medicine are eligible for these programs. All 18 CPEP training programs typically have 1 fellow and some have 2 fellows. Three institutions have both ACGME and CPEP fellows. Graduates of CPEP programs are eligible to take the American Board of Medical Microbiology (ABMM) certification examination.

The third option is to certify through the American Board of Bioanalysis (ABB) as a High Complexity Laboratory Director (HCLD). Individuals eligible to take this certification examination must have an earned doctoral degree in the life sciences or chemistry and 4 years of technical experience. It also qualifies them to direct CLIA-approved high-complexity laboratories. Individuals who pass any of these 3 board examinations are eligible for licensure as laboratory directors in states requiring it.

The CDC in conjunction with the Association of Public Health Laboratories has developed a new program called Laboratory Leadership Service that is patterned after the Epidemic Intelligence Service. The purpose of this program that began in 2015 is to train doctoral-level scientists for leadership roles in public health laboratories. Two-year experiential training in State Public Health and CDC Laboratories is the major focus of this program. Individuals eligible to apply are those with an earned doctorate in a laboratory-related discipline and who have 2 years of postdoctoral experience preferably in a discipline broadly related to public health. Based on current eligibility criteria, individuals completing this program would not be eligible for any of the 3 certification examinations, although with appropriate experience, they would be eligible for both the ABB's HCLD and the ABMM certification examinations.

HOW TO ATTRACT THE NEXT GENERATION OF CLINICAL MICROBIOLOGIST?

Probably the greatest challenge in attracting the next generation of clinical microbiologists is that they are part of an "invisible army" of health care workers who are virtually unknown to the general public.[23] Although there is great emphasis on Science, Technology, Engineering and Mathematics (STEM) education in the United States because it is deemed to be where great future career opportunity lies, medical laboratory science is not listed on STEM career Web sites[29] despite the fact that compensation is improving, although still not at the level of other health care–related careers,[32] and opportunities are abundant. A new approach begun in the fall of 2018 at the authors' university is to offer a 1-hour pass-fail course that exposes prehealth students to different medical careers, including medical laboratory science. One rationale for the course is that students who do not have a competitive academic record for medical, dental, or pharmacy school may find satisfying careers in other health disciplines if they knew about them. In its first 2 semesters, it has attracted more than 600 students. It is hoped this class will help attract an increasing number of people to alternate health care–related careers, including medical laboratory science.

Because the current and future generations are "wired," using venues like YouTube, Instagram, Twitter, and blogs might be an important way to inform individuals about careers in clinical microbiology. The American Society for Microbiology is using all of these approaches to try to attract individuals to the microbial sciences. How successful that will be in attracting individuals to medical laboratory science with a specific interest in clinical microbiology is currently unknown.

Supervisors and managers come almost exclusively from the ranks of bench-level technologists, so recruitment in that area is primarily dependent on getting young people interested in medical laboratory science as a career path.

The authors have had a medical microbiology training program at their institution for more than 40 years. One of the most encouraging recent trends is a significant expansion in the applicant pool for this program. In this decade, pools of 20 to 30 applicants per position have expanded to 75 to 100 applicants per position with a concomitant increase in applicant quality. PhD students are recognizing that the traditional route of becoming a professor with government grants is becoming an increasingly difficult career path. They have found CPEP training programs to offer an excellent alternative.[23]

HOW TO TRAIN THEM?

Currently there are 234 MLS and 244 MLT programs in the United States that between them graduated close to 7000 individuals in 2017.[29] A key feature of medical laboratory science education at the associate, bachelor, and master levels is experiential learning. Experience down through the years suggests this is an effective approach to training individuals for bench-level jobs in the clinical microbiology laboratory. Apprentice types of education programs, like the one pioneered by UCLA that also concentrates on experiential learning, are also proving to be successful. Another novel approach is an online course leading to a master's degree in clinical microbiology that has been developed by George Washington University but requires a practicum that can be challenging for the student to find near where he or she lives. A further barrier in this program is that the student is responsible for arranging his or her clinical rotation.

There are 4 significant challenges that need to be addressed in the initial and ongoing training of clinical microbiologists, as follows:

1. How do individuals who are trained in automated laboratories get appropriate experiential training that prepares them to work in laboratories that are not extensively automated? Although at first glance this may seem to be a significant problem, basic microbiology principles still apply regardless of the technology available in the laboratory. For microbial cultures, MLS and MLT must still be able to read plates and know basic phenotypic characteristics of common organisms.[33] They must also be able to interpret microbial stains and recognize clinically significant findings, especially critical values. Perhaps the biggest challenge is students who train in the laboratory using mass spectroscopy for the bulk of organism identifications who then find themselves in a laboratory that uses automated identification systems, such as Vitek or MicroScan, to identify organisms. Again, basic principles apply. Do the organism's culture characteristics match its identification? Does this unusual organism identification make sense in the clinical setting? Developing these analytical skills is essential during training. One of the areas that is lacking in training MLS and MLT students is how to interpret the scientific literature. Because there are so many "new" scientific journals, many of which are open access, for profit of dubious quality referred to as "predatory" journals, it is important that MLSs and MLTs understand certain basic principles, such as the principle of sensitivity, specificity, positive and negative predictive values, and inherent bias in the data being presented.
2. How do we train individuals to work as a team member in a technologically complex medical system with increasing complex clinical microbiology data that they will need to help the clinician interpret? As mentioned previously, medical education is putting much less emphasis on basic science knowledge,[24] resulting in significant gaps in knowledge among clinicians. The bench level technologist becomes the first line to educate and assist the clinician in understanding complex clinical microbiology data. The challenge is to train the bench MLSs and MLTs to be comfortable with explaining "routine" information, such as methicillin-resistant *Staphylococcus aureus* is resistant to all beta-lactams, but make them aware if asked by the physician, "What drug should I use?" to consult with the hospital's pharmacists or infectious disease clinicians. The bench MLSs and MLTs should also recognize when they should consult with the laboratory specialist, supervisor, or director for more complex issues.

3. Clinical microbiology knowledge is rapidly increasing at a time when workforce limitations make it difficult to find time for traditional continuing education at off-site locales given at fixed times. One of the essentials for success in any medically related career is to be a life-long learner. Given the amount of information that is available electronically, it is important that individuals learn how to find reliable information. The authors' approach has been to make clear to their technical staff what they believe to be reliable sources of information. The authors would include the CDC Web site, Clinical and Laboratory Standards Institute (CLSI) documents, infectious disease society of america (IDSA) and american society for mirobiology (ASM) clinical practice guidelines, and the Manual of Clinical Microbiology. The authors also encourage their technologists to use PubMed to determine the clinical significance of unusual organisms. Importantly, all these resources are available in the authors' laboratory with most of them available electronically at their work stations. It certainly would be beneficial if a clinical microbiology "Up-to-Date" could be developed by the American Society for Microbiology. Brief (7–15 minute) continuing education programs available online would also be useful for the life-long learner. As previously mentioned, selected TED Talks and YouTube videos are a good model for this approach. The College of American Pathology offers a competency program for clinical laboratories that also provides access to continuing education credits that technologists can use to renew their board certifications.

4. For manager/supervisors, most of the institutional training is focused on basic supervisory/manager courses in human resources. The assumption is that because the individual came up through "the ranks," that they were chosen for the management position in large part because of their excellent time management and leadership skills along with superior technical abilities. However, to be effective at strategic planning, an essential skill at this level, the individual must continue to enhance their scientific knowledge fund. How this can best be accomplished is currently an open question.

The 2 postdoctoral training programs, ACGME and CPEP, have a standardized curriculum and a strong experiential training component. In the authors' experience with their CPEP program, the following 3 aspects stand out and are essential for training doctoral level scientists:

1. High-level experiential training, where the fellow learns to perform genomic and proteomic analysis, especially troubleshooting problems inherent in these technologies.
2. Daily interaction with the health care team, especially infectious disease physicians and pharmacists, allows the trainee to learn the language of medicine, allowing effective communication with clinicians; to develop clinical problems solving skills; and to recognize gaps in diagnostic technologies.
3. Development of analytical and research skills that will allow them to address the clinical microbiology challenges of tomorrow.

SUMMARY

Infectious disease diagnostics is rapidly advancing and changing. In order for these advances to be translated into improved patient care, a well-trained workforce composed of life-long learners is essential. Our discipline needs to attract talented, motivated individuals to the opportunities that are clearly available. Experience has shown us that there is a pool of individuals interested in microbiology and working in health care settings, but they have no idea what education is needed accomplish this. It is incumbent upon the clinical microbiology community to educate young people about these opportunities and show them the career path available to them. Someone helped us identify this important, satisfying career; we need to help others.

REFERENCES

1. Renner ED, Gatheridge LA, Washington JA 2nd. Evaluation of radiometric system for detecting bacteremia. Appl Microbiol 1973;26:368–72.
2. Prevost E, Bannister E. Detection of yeast septicemia by biphasic and radiometric methods. J Clin Microbiol 1981;13:655–60.
3. Truant AL, Starr E, Nevel CA, et al. Comparison of AMS-Vitek, MicroScan, and Autobac series II for the identification of gram-negative bacilli. Diagn Microbiol Infect Dis 1989;12:211–5.
4. Payne WJ Jr, Marshall DL, Shockley RK, et al. Clinical laboratory applications of monoclonal antibodies. Clin Microbiol Rev 1988;1:313–29.
5. Thorpe TC, Wilson ML, Turner JE, et al. BacT/Alert: an automated colorimetric microbial detection system. J Clin Microbiol 1990;28:1608–12.
6. Mullis KB. The unusual origin of the polymerase chain reaction. Sci Am 1990;262:56–61, 64–5.
7. Espy MJ, Uhl JR, Sloan LM, et al. Real-time PCR in clinical microbiology: applications for routine laboratory testing. Clin Microbiol Rev 2006;19:165–256.
8. Hodinka RL. Point: is the era of viral culture over in the clinical microbiology laboratory? J Clin Microbiol 2013;51:2–4.
9. Ramanan P, Bryson AL, Binnicker MJ, et al. Syndromic panel-based testing in clinical microbiology. Clin Microbiol Rev 2018;31 [pii:e00024-17].
10. Dien Bard J, Alby K. Point-counterpoint: meningitis/encephalitis syndromic testing in the clinical laboratory. J Clin Microbiol 2018;56 [pii:e00018-18].
11. Chiu CY. Viral pathogen discovery. Curr Opin Microbiol 2013;16:468–78.
12. Quainoo S, Coolen JPM, van Hijum S, et al. Whole-genome sequencing of bacterial pathogens: the future of nosocomial outbreak analysis. Clin Microbiol Rev 2017;30:1015–63.
13. Taur Y, Pamer EG. Harnessing microbiota to kill a pathogen: fixing the microbiota to treat Clostridium difficile infections. Nat Med 2014;20:246–7.
14. Huang YJ, LiPuma JJ. The microbiome in cystic fibrosis. Clin Chest Med 2016;37:59–67.
15. Clark AE, Kaleta EJ, Arora A, et al. Matrix-assisted laser desorption ionization-time of flight mass spectrometry: a fundamental shift in the routine practice of clinical microbiology. Clin Microbiol Rev 2013;26:547–603.
16. Tran A, Alby K, Kerr A, et al. Cost savings realized by implementation of routine microbiological identification by matrix-assisted laser desorption ionization-time of flight mass spectrometry. J Clin Microbiol 2015;53:2473–9.
17. Garcia E, Kundu I, Ali A, et al. The American Society for Clinical Pathology's 2016-2017 vacancy survey of medical laboratories in the United States. Am J Clin Pathol 2018;149:387–400.
18. Bailey A, Ledeboer N, Burnham CD. Clinical microbiology is growing up: the total laboratory automation revolution. Clin Chem 2018. https://doi.org/10.1373/clinchem.2017.274522.
19. Thomson RB Jr, McElvania E. Blood culture results reporting: how fast is your laboratory and is faster better? J Clin Microbiol 2018;56:e01313-8.

20. Theparee T, Das S, Thomson RB Jr. Total laboratory automation and matrix-assisted laser desorption ionization-time of flight mass spectrometry improve turnaround times in the clinical microbiology laboratory: a retrospective analysis. J Clin Microbiol 2018;56 [pii:e01242-17].
21. Tabak YP, Vankeepuram L, Ye G, et al. Blood culture turnaround time in U.S. Acute care hospitals and implications for laboratory process optimization. J Clin Microbiol 2018;56:e00500–18.
22. Brecher SM. Waltzing around sacred cows on the way to the future. J Clin Microbiol 2018;56 [pii:e01779-17].
23. Gilligan PH. The invisible army. J Clin Microbiol 2017;55:2583–9.
24. Naritoku WY, Vasovic L, Steinberg JJ, et al. Anatomic and clinical pathology boot camps: filling pathology-specific gaps in undergraduate medical education. Arch Pathol Lab Med 2014;138:316–21.
25. Perry JD. A decade of development of chromogenic culture media for clinical microbiology in an era of molecular diagnostics. Clin Microbiol Rev 2017;30:449–79.
26. Plebani M. Errors in clinical laboratories or errors in laboratory medicine? Clin Chem Lab Med 2006;44:750–9.
27. Schultz K, Sickbert-Bennett E, Marx A, et al. Preventable patient harm: a multidisciplinary, bundled approach to reducing Clostridium difficile infections while using a glutamate dehydrogenase/toxin immunochromatographic assay/nucleic acid amplification test diagnostic algorithm. J Clin Microbiol 2018;56 [pii: e00625-18].
28. Flores AL, Risley K, Quintana K. Developing a public health pipeline: key components of a public health leadership program. Prev Med Community Health 2018. [Epub ahead of print].
29. ASCLS. Addressing the clinical laboratory workforce shortage. Chicago (IL): The American Society for Clinical Laboratory Science; 2018.
30. American Society for Clinical Pathology. The medical laboratory personnel shortage (policy number 04-04) 2018.
31. Chandrasekar P, Havkichek D, Johnson LB. Infectious disease subspeciality: declining demand challenges and opportunities. Clin Infect Dis 2014;59:1593–8.
32. Medical Laboratory Observer. MLO's 2018 annual salary survey of laboratory professionals 2018.
33. Clinical and Laboratory Standards Institute. M35-A2 abbreviated identification of bacteria and yeast; approved guideline. 2nd edition 2008.

We Cannot Do It Alone
The Intersection of Public Health, Public Policy, and Clinical Microbiology

Rose A. Lee, MD, MSPH[a,b,c,d], James E. Kirby, MD, D(ABMM)[b,e,*]

KEYWORDS

- Public health microbiology • Epidemiology • FoodNet
- Antimicrobial Resistant Laboratory Network • FDA-CDC Biobank
- Laboratory-developed test • New antibiotics • Multidrug resistance

KEY POINTS

- National resources such as the FDA-CDC AR Isolate Bank can support clinical laboratories at a local level as they confront multidrug-resistant pathogens and should be supported, strengthened, and expanded.
- Distributed networks such as the Antimicrobial Resistance Laboratory Network offer specialized diagnostics to address specific needs such as unconventional antimicrobial susceptibility testing not yet available at a local level.
- Public resources should be made available to help laboratories develop and standardize tests to address pressing infectious disease diagnostic needs that are not commercially compelling for assay development.
- Continuously updated local, regional, and national antibiograms should be available to guide therapeutic decisions with granularity and guide public health interventions.
- Policies and regulations should balance reliability of laboratory testing with fostering rapid entrance of infectious diagnostics into the market.

Disclosure Statement: J.E. Kirby is a member of the Clinical Advisory Board of First Light Biosciences, Chelmsford, MA. TECAN (Morrisville, NC) provided an HP D300 digital dispenser and associated consumables used by J.E. Kirby's research group during development of rapid and at-will antimicrobial susceptibility testing diagnostics. Neither First Light nor TECAN had a role in article preparation or decision to publish.

[a] Department of Pathology, Beth Israel Deaconess Medical Center, Center for Life Science, 3 Blackfan Circle – CLS 5th FL 517/4C, Boston, MA 02115, USA; [b] Harvard Medical School, Boston, MA, USA; [c] Division of Infectious Diseases, Department of Medicine, Beth Israel Deaconess Medical Center, Boston, MA, USA; [d] Department of Pediatrics, Boston Children's Hospital, Boston, MA, USA; [e] Clinical Microbiology, Department of Pathology, Beth Israel Deaconess Medical Center, 330 Brookline Avenue - YA309, Boston, MA, USA
* Corresponding author. Beth Israel Deaconess Medical Center, Department of Pathology, 330 Brookline Avenue - YA309, Boston, MA, USA.
E-mail address: jekirby@bidmc.harvard.edu
; @kirbylabmicrobe (J.E.K.)

INTRODUCTION

The intersection of public health with clinical microbiology has been apparent since John Snow established the connection of cholera with the Broad Street pump. As we have been challenged by communicable disease crises from the human immuno-deficiency virus (HIV) epidemic to the rise of carbapenem-resistant Enterobacteri-aceae (CRE), our society has amassed new tools to diagnose and treat these infections. Nevertheless, with evolving resistance and emerging infections, the urgent need to fight such threats in a coordinated fashion at a local and societal level con-tinues. The authors therefore review microbiological public health resources and stra-tegies, and reflect on policies needed to combat microbial threats of the future.

NATIONAL RESOURCES AVAILABLE AT LOCAL LEVEL

Bringing new drugs on board: new antibiotics offer potentially life-saving options for multidrug-resistant infections. However, they are only useful clinically if the microbi-ology laboratory can provide timely antimicrobial susceptibility testing (AST) results. Historically there has been a time lag in the availability of susceptibility testing methods for new antibiotics. As a result, isolates must be sent to a reference labora-tory delaying AST results for up to a week or more. However, for an AST result to be meaningful for patient management, it usually must be available in a few days at most.

In the recent past, the time delay between Food and Drug Administration (FDA) approval of new antimicrobials and the availability of corresponding AST methods has been a significant hindrance to the utilization of new drugs for clinical care. Cef-taroline, for example, did not have an FDA-cleared AST method until 7 months after the initial approval in 2010 and automated systems took another 2.5 to 3.5 years to gain clearance. The FDA recognized this problematic discordance and hence made efforts to coordinate release of antimicrobials and commercial AST methods.[1] Howev-er, it can still take years before novel antimicrobials become incorporated into com-mercial panels. Fortunately, diffusion-based methods may offer an interim solution.

Nevertheless, before implementation of any AST method for a new drug, clinical lab-oratories must still verify its performance per Clinical Laboratory Improvement Amend-ments (CLIA) of 1988 requirement. CLIA stipulations are nonspecific and for FDA-approved assays only indicate the need to verify accuracy and precision to an un-stated degree. In the absence of explicit guidance, use of accepted standards in the field are a reasonable and commonly used substitute, codified in documents such as Cumitech 31A.[2]

Verification could entail comparing the new AST method with a reference standard such as broth microdilution (BMD), but this gold-standard method requires significant assay expertise, technologist effort, and ready availability of antimicrobial powder. Most hospital laboratories consequently opt to verify new AST methods using a set of strains already characterized by a reference method such as BMD (or a nonrefer-ence, FDA-cleared method that has been previously verified in a CLIA-accredited lab-oratory) and that has an appropriate representation of susceptible and resistant isolates.

Practically, for new antibiotics, where to find such characterized strain sets is un-clear. Availability of appropriate strains sets is also needed for "off-label" verification of existing methods when breakpoints are adjusted to reflect evolving best practice consensus (eg, annual Clinical and Laboratory Standards Institute updates). The often-recommended fall back for the latter is to compare with the disk diffusion method using correspondingly updated zone sizes.[3] The rationale is that the disk diffu-sion method for common drugs was instituted before CLIA 1988 and therefore is exempt from its own verification requirements,[4] a somewhat problematic strategy, as the disks were originally cleared based on categorical performance around former, but not updated breakpoints, and accordingly important essential agreement metrics cannot be assessed.

Obviously for new drugs, appropriate, well-characterized strain sets must be possessed by pharmaceutical manufacturers or affiliates, as data from these strains are required to establish the susceptibility breakpoints for the drug. Under current regulations, however, pharmaceutical companies are prohibited from proactively either providing or sourcing characterized strains sets for clinical laboratories. Oddly, clinical laboratories can independently inquire on a need-to-know basis, freeing pharmaceutical companies to reveal some potential options. Such obstructive policies should be remedied by governing bodies, as the ability for clinical laboratories to verify, and thereby enable clinicians to use novel antimicrobials, is just as important as their commercial availability.

The FDA-Centers for Disease Control and Prevention *(CDC) Antimicrobial Resistance Isolate Bank*: fortunately, the FDA-CDC Antimicrobial Resistance (AR) Isolate Bank now provides a way to circumvent this conundrum. Launched in July 2015 as a tool to combat antimicrobial resistance, this highly valuable public health resource provides a curated repository of genotypically and phenotypically characterized bacterial isolates with clinically important resistance mechanisms and reference minimum inhibitory concentrations (MICs) to novel and standard antimicrobials.[5,6]

The FDA-CDC AR Isolate Bank is a paradigm of a public health resource that supports clinical laboratories at a local level to provide potentially life-saving, rapid, and up-to-date AST reporting. For example, the AR Isolate Bank includes an *Enterobacteriaceae* carbapenem breakpoint panel designed to assist with verification and implementation of new Clinical and Laboratory Standards Institute (CLSI) carbapenem breakpoints, given emergence of novel resistance mechanisms. The gram-negative carbapenemase detection panel supports verification of tests for carbapenemase production such as the modified carbapenem inactivation method (mCIM) and EDTA-mCIM (eCIM), which can distinguish serine β-lactamases from metallo-β-lactamases.[7] Importantly, these strain sets include an assortment of well-characterized multidrug-resistance mechanisms, such as a range of serine and metallo-carbapenemases, which would be difficult for clinical laboratories to collect comprehensively from their own patients or purchase, and thereby allow clinical laboratories to gain experience with detection of critical resistance elements in their own laboratories.

Extending this idea further, imagine strain sets distributed widely to clinical laboratories for which curated modal MIC data for each new antibiotic would be released coincident with FDA approval. Analogously, as CLSI updates breakpoints, including changes such as new susceptible dose-dependent (SDD) categories to address emerging resistance patterns, there would ideally be concomitant AR Isolate Bank deployment of strain sets with modal MICs within and bordering the relevant MIC ranges to aid laboratories in verifying and promptly adopting these revisions. Particularly in the superbug era, accurate AST reporting of SDD categories formerly classified as "intermediate" can be crucial in providing appropriate salvage therapeutic options for multidrug resistant infections.[8]

In summary, the recently created FDA-CDC AR Isolate Bank provides welcome support for clinical microbiology laboratories as well as a resource for researchers, diagnostics, and pharmaceutical companies. This resource should be supported and strengthened, and ongoing "free availability" should be maintained with release/ updating of panels to coincide with new drug approvals to counterbalance disincentives for clinical laboratories and companies to invest in capacity for rarely used antimicrobials and testing.

Dare we ask? We also might consider, if new AST methods were appropriately vetted by the FDA, the encore verification performance by clinical laboratories, whether limited or extensive, seems superfluous. It is estimated to take approximately 2 days of technologist and director time to validate a new E-test or disk method with 30 to 40 strains—that is, a discouraging barrier for bringing new AST tests on board. Importantly, laboratories also perform a mini-verification every time they perform a test by running quality control (QC) testing with confirmation that results are within specified limits (individualized QC plan, exceptions aside). Presumably QC requirements are deemed appropriately discriminatory for evaluation of ongoing assay performance, so why the initial extra verification step? Verification should be an issue for initial vetting by the manufacturer with appropriately large, representative strain sets, and test product deficits should not fall under the purview of postmarketing discovery by laboratories with greatly differing capabilities. If this seemingly redundant and purposefully vague verification requirement were lifted, the broad array of AST testing for new drugs could be implemented within days! Another option, although potentially burdensome and perhaps unnecessary, would be to task a set of high complexity clinical laboratories on a volunteer basis or possibly with some financial recompense to perform an independent assessment to verify manufacturer's claims that could be relied on by the field.

Antimicrobial Resistance Laboratory Network (ARLN): with emerging multidrug resistance, clinical laboratories are more frequently encountering pathogens for which there are no active agents based on routine or even reference laboratory-based AST. Although novel antimicrobials in clinical trials may be available on a compassionate-use basis, existing agents used in combination regimens are worthy of consideration as well. For example, aztreonam, a monobactam, remains active against metallo-carbapenemases such as the New Delhi metallo-β-lactamase 1, and ceftazidime-avibactam provides activity against AmpC and extended-spectrum- β-lactamases (ESBLs), which are enzymes that inactivate aztreonam. Accordingly, a regimen that inhibits AmpC and ESBL degradation of aztreonam, which then can function in the presence of potent metallo-carbapenemases should be active against "superbugs" carrying these dangerous resistance elements.[9] However, the question remains how a clinical laboratory would determine whether combinatorial salvage regimens are active against a given isolate.

The CDC has recently set up the ARLN to offer such testing. Established in 2016, the ARLN is composed of 7 regional laboratories and the National Tuberculosis Molecular Surveillance Center where clinical laboratories around the United States can send resistant isolates for additional testing. Their laboratory network has adopted inkjet printing technology for this AST testing, originally described by Smith and Kirby and Brennan-Krohn and Kirby, that allows highly accurate and precise at-will set-up and testing of any desired antimicrobial alone or in combination with reference broth microdilution equivalent AST results.[10–14] The ALRN currently offers, for example, the combination AST of aztreonam + ceftazidime-avibactam. Furthermore, it has the capacity to characterize isolates via whole genome sequencing and other molecular testing. Most importantly, the ARLN provides a distributed laboratory network that brings new AST and surveillance capabilities closer to the point of patient care. Alternatively, in the future, equivalent technology and antimicrobial reagents could and should be deployed at referral hospitals where superbugs are more prevalent.

Central data and analyte repositories to support laboratory-developed test (LDT) design and validation: there has been little industry interest in commercializing and seeking FDA approval for molecular diagnostics for clinically important yet less common infectious diseases. LDTs fill this unmet need. LDTs are in vitro diagnostic tests developed and verified for local use. FDA-cleared methods that have been modified in any way by a clinical microbiology laboratory are also considered LDTs.[2]

Prominent examples of LDTs would include viral load testing for BK virus, Epstein-Barr virus, and cytomegalovirus (CMV) in the transplant setting. Although there are FDA-cleared assays for CMV viral load testing in blood, testing in other specimen types such as bronchoalveolar lavage, urine, and saliva provide added value for certain populations. Application of revised breakpoints to existing commercial AST methods are also considered a modification and therefore an LDT. Commercial manufacturers often take years to seek clearance for such updates, as the FDA does not have the authority to require companies to submit data within a certain timeframe. Accordingly, during this interval, clinical laboratories must verify accuracy and precision across revised breakpoints. Without the capacity or expertise to implement LDTs, laboratories presumably must continue to use outdated breakpoints, which could miss resistant strains and undermine patient care. As one example of the magnitude of this issue, 28% of laboratories in California had not yet lowered carbapenem breakpoints within 5 years of CLSI introducing revised, evidenced-based cutoffs in 2010.[15] Alternatively, LDT testing, whether for molecular diagnosis of target pathogens or AST determinations with revised breakpoints, may be performed at reference laboratories, which have extensive menus of LDTs but with suboptimal turnaround time delays.

There is ongoing debate about the appropriate level of regulation required for LDTs and whether routine laboratory quality assurance activities under CLIA 1988 are sufficient. Given the rapid growth of LDTs in personalized medicine, the American Society for Clinical Pathology recommended that "the regulatory infrastructure adopted must be sufficiently meticulous to safeguard the public without being so burdensome that it impedes emerging technology."[16] As a comparator, in Europe most diagnostic tests are considered low-risk and exempt from premarket evaluation. Therefore, clinical quality of LDTs is managed through professionally driven quality assessment infrastructure.[16] The authors agree with this latter approach.

By analogy to the FDA-CDC AR Isolate Bank, the authors envision a public health resource to assist in LDT development that would have the added benefit of greater standardization of assays between institutions. Currently, microbiology laboratories independently construct and validate LDTs for similar sets of pathogens, given comparable clinical needs and the lack of commercial testing options. A free centralized publicly available database of pooled procedural and validation information would provide a much more comprehensive understanding of assay design and performance and allow laboratories to benefit from collective experience instead of each reinventing the wheel on its own. Best practice procedures including reagent and assay performance characteristics could then be described in consensus guidelines, which would ultimately increase the quality of overall diagnostic testing.

An expansion of interinstitutional comparable LDTs would also significantly bolster surveillance programs, as smaller facilities that otherwise may not have had the technical expertise to adopt LDTs may now be able to contribute to the nationwide diagnostic capacity to understand important microbiological concerns such as spread of viral subtypes, sexually transmitted infections, or antimicrobial resistance. To expand this idea further, the authors also propose a repository of free publicly available critical analytes that would allow standardization of LDT assays across facilities (eg, viral load standards) and ensure robust detection, for example, of critical viral subtypes in the face of genetic drift and emerging variants.

IT IS TIME TO ADOPT A DIFFERENT MODEL FOR DIAGNOSTIC TEST APPROVAL IN AREAS OF UNMET MEDICAL NEED

An alternative and bolder strategy would be to lower the regulatory burden for approval of infectious disease diagnostics in areas of unmet need. Our proposal would be to lower the approval threshold for areas of focused need that would not normally be appealing for commercial development under current regulations. Specifically, companies would still have to establish robust analytical performance for their methodology, however, without the need for extensive and costly clinical trials to establish clinical performance/utility. This would spur innovation, development, and implementation of laboratory tests in areas such as detection of rare emerging diseases (MERS, Ebola, carbapenemase detection and discrimination, blood parasites, seasonal influenza subtyping for therapeutic discrimination, tick-borne bloodstream infection, and *Candida auris* to forestall hospital outbreaks). Transplant and immunocompromised host infectious disease testing could also be extended to the range of sample types of importance (eg, bronchoalveolar lavage fluid and other respiratory specimens for molecular detection of Pneumocystis jiroveci pneumonia (PJP) and toxoplasma among others). The European diagnostics market, for example, offers excellent diagnostic support for clinical care without the extra layer of regulatory burden.

Freed of the need to determine clinical validity, companies could confirm analytical performance in multiple sample types, thereby in turn freeing clinical laboratories from replicative efforts to develop LDTs when existing testing platforms would suffice. Those companies that could offer testing on the multitude of sample types of interest would have a competitive advantage, and competition would then spur a comprehensive testing menu to the benefit of the patients.

Furthermore, the demand for expensive reference laboratory testing would be decreased and more timely local diagnosis would reduce inefficiencies in the health care system, avoid unnecessary expense-associated delayed diagnosis, and contribute positively to patient well-being. The authors therefore encourage a rethinking of current regulatory framework in the United States. For areas of unmet need, we should put decision-making capability about clinical utility into the hands of medical specialists (laboratory medicine/clinical microbiology/infectious diseases) who can evaluate the most up-to-date medical and scientific literature in concert with evaluation of analytical performance capabilities, published in product inserts and vetted by the FDA, and make appropriate decisions about assays and platforms.

Setting the standard: strong national and international standards for quality assurance, method performance, and interpretative criteria should be strengthened and maintained. The authors acknowledge the contribution of both national and international organizations such as CLSI, EUCAST (European Committee on Antimicrobial Susceptibility Testing), USCAST (United States Committee on Antimicrobial Susceptibility Testing), SIS (Swedish Standards Institute), CEN (European Committee for Standardization), and ISO (International Organization of Standardization) that establish such standards. Many are volunteer-driven, membership- and/or government-supported not-for-profit entities. The authors also applaud coordination between organizations such as the FDA and CLSI. They encourage their continued, proactive review of breakpoints based on the most current understanding of pharmacokinetics and pharmacodynamics, which may suggest revisiting of values established during original drug approval.

STRENGTHENING PUBLIC HEALTH LABORATORY SURVEILLANCE

National surveillance programs represent a key intersection between public health and microbiology laboratories. One of the oldest examples is the Foodborne Diseases

Active Surveillance Network (FoodNet), established in 1995 as a collaboration between 10 state health departments, that monitors for significant infectious enteric pathogens.[17] FoodNet determines the burden and trends in foodborne illness in order to appropriately design prevention and intervention programs.

Several other CDC surveillance systems for tracking food and waterborne diseases include Foodborne Disease Outbreak Surveillance System (FDOSS), National Antimicrobial Resistance Monitoring System for Enteric Bacteria (NARMS), and Waterborne Disease and Outbreak Surveillance (WBDOSS) among others.[18] Although certain programs function more closely with Infection Control and Epidemiology departments to gather relevant patient clinical data, all of these systems require interaction with the microbiology laboratory for appropriate identification and isolate collection.

Some of the programs such as PulseNet provide bacterial DNA fingerprinting (previously pulsed-field gel electrophoresis now transitioning to whole genome sequencing) of foodborne illnesses. This data revolutionized epidemic investigations, because outbreaks could be identified and intervened on in hours to days instead of weeks in the previous era when epidemiologists had to wait for new patients to meet appropriate case criteria in order to identify clinical patterns that suggest a novel outbreak[19].

The need for shared surveillance and diagnostic data repositories has been recognized among international collaborations as well. TBnet is one illustration of a partnership of European pulmonologists, epidemiologists, and infectious disease specialists organized on the premise of shared research goals, with a particular interest in immunodiagnostic tools. They accordingly have developed their own TB Biobank in addition to a data repository using common collection methods to simplify cross-study comparison.[20]

Similarly, the Program for Monitoring Emerging Diseases (ProMED-mail) is an entity founded in 1994 and maintained by the International Society of Infectious Diseases. Conceived as a free Internet listserv tool for rapid detection and report of emerging infectious or toxin-mediated diseases, ProMED-mail expanded from only 40 subscribers at its inception to greater than 83,000 in more than 150 countries. Subscribers receive e-mail reports filtered and moderated by a specialist panel on outbreaks and disease emergence. ProMED-mail voiced the earliest public account of severe acute respiratory syndrome and warned the medical community throughout the world of this outbreak.[21,22]

In this era of globalization with common threats and pathogens facing individual hospitals, states, and nations, it makes intuitive sense that these efforts to collect and share data should be fostered and strengthened.

Information exchange: real-time publicly available data to track infectious diseases is essential to control and prevent efforts and ever more relevant as demonstrated by ProMED-mail's internet-based success. FluNet is a model prototype that should be extrapolated to other emerging infectious threats. Established in 1997, FluNet is a global web-based data collection and reporting tool for influenza and logs viruses by subtype with records updated weekly.[23] SENTRY and ATLAS provide worldwide tracking of AST data for currently available antimicrobials.[24,25]

Expanded surveillance programs that, for example, track CRE by genotype should be public health goals achievable with current bioinformatic platforms. As one example of potential impact, the Israel National Center for Infection Control initiated an effort in 2008 within long-term care facilities where they collected a real-time database of all CRE carriers and events leading to acquisition. The program facilitated supervised information exchange and encompassed approximately 25,000 beds over 300 institutions enabling early detection of carriers and implementation of population-specific contact precautions.[26] These efforts achieved more than a 10-fold reduction of CRE point prevalence in their acute hospital network and 50% reduction in all facilities. There is no doubt that such efforts will become increasingly important as new resistance emerges.

Annually updated hospital-based antibiograms are insufficient to guide empirical therapy with emerging antimicrobial resistance. Automated, deidentified input from hospital and laboratory information systems that provide regional to national metadata to track and forecast patterns of antibiotic resistance is a reasonable goal for our public health infrastructure. Daily updated facility; regional, national, and international (for travelers) species; and clone-specific antibiograms should be available to guide empirical therapeutic choice. Integration with whole-genome sequencing will facilitate clone tracking, illuminate resistance evolution, and inform local and public health countermeasures. As sources of new epidemics, infections, and/or resistance may be identified, there may be local opposition to participation. However, with balanced levels of access by health care providers and the public, the overarching public good of this early detection and control infrastructure should outweigh economic disincentives.

SUMMARY

Microbiological data are necessary to inform public health goals and strategies, and conversely public health goals help guide the diagnostic strategies pursued in laboratories. In an era of rising global infectious disease threats, the public health laboratory infrastructure requires maintenance and strengthening to forestall harm to individual patients and populations. A pressing public health and societal need is the framework and infrastructure to streamline adoption of new antimicrobials and diagnostics. We analogously need streamlined, real-time output from the microbiology laboratories with centralized data aggregation to detect spread of resistant organisms and direct appropriate local and public health countermeasures. Here, the authors review some of the major existing resources that have supported our public health efforts and also identify programs and policies that could be of significant benefit. Governments, standards organizations, researchers, industry, and clinical microbiology laboratories should continue to collaborate to better address unmet public health goals and individual needs of infected patients.

ACKNOWLEDGMENTS

Based on space limitations, it was not possible for us to reference and cite all of the relevant literature in the public health field related to clinical microbiology and necessarily were selective. We thank Kenneth P. Smith for helpful comments on the article. The author Dr. R.A. Lee was supported by the Eunice Kennedy Shriver National Institute of Child Health and Human Development of the National Institutes of Health pediatric infectious diseases research training grant, T32HD055148. The content is solely the responsibility of the authors and does not necessarily represent the official views of the National Institutes of Health.

REFERENCES

1. Humphries RM, Kircher S, Ferrell A, et al. The continued value of disk diffusion for assessing antimicrobial susceptibility in clinical laboratories: report from the clinical and laboratory standards Institute methods development and standardization working group. J Clin Microbiol 2018;56(8) [pii:e00437-18].

2. Clark RB, Lewisnski ML, Loeffelholtz MJ, et al. Verification and validation of procedures in the clinical microbiology laboratory. In: Sharp SE, editor. Cumitech, vol. 31A. Washington, DC: American Society of Microbiology; 2009.
3. Infectious Diseases Society of America. A minimal validation study for application of revised CLSI beta-lactam breakpoints to interpret lower range MICs Generated by a commercial susceptibility Device. ISDA Practice Guidelines. 2018. Available at: https://www.idsociety.org/globalassets/idsa/topics-of-interest/antimicrobial-resistance/appendix-a-brief-validation-protocol-final.pdf. Accessed April 23, 2019.
4. Heil EL, Johnson JK. Impact of CLSI breakpoint changes on microbiology laboratories and antimicrobial stewardship programs. J Clin Microbiol 2016;54(4): 840–4.
5. CDC & FDA antibiotic resistance (AR) Isolate Bank. US Centers for disease control and prevention. Available at: https://www.cdc.gov/drugresistance/resistance-bank/index.html. Accessed April 5, 2019.
6. Lutgring JD, Machado MJ, Benahmed FH, et al. FDA-CDC antimicrobial resistance Isolate Bank: a publicly available resource to support research, development, and regulatory requirements. J Clin Microbiol 2018;56(2) [pii:e01415-17].
7. CLSI. Performance standards for antimicrobial suceptibility testing— 28th Edition. CLSI Supplement M100. Wayne (PA): Clinical and Laboratory Standards Institute; 2018. p. 108–18.
8. Smith KP, Brennan-Krohn T, Weir S, et al. Improved accuracy of cefepime susceptibility testing for extended-spectrum-beta-lactamase-producing Enterobacteriaceae with an on-demand digital dispensing method. J Clin Microbiol 2017; 55(2):470–8.
9. Marshall S, Hujer AM, Rojas LJ, et al. Can ceftazidime-avibactam and aztreonam overcome beta-lactam resistance conferred by metallo-beta-lactamases in enterobacteriaceae? Antimicrob Agents Chemother 2017;61(4) [pii:e02243-16].
10. Brennan-Krohn T, Kirby JE. Antimicrobial synergy testing by the inkjet printer-assisted automated checkerboard array and the manual time-kill method. J Vis Exp 2019;146:e58636.
11. Brennan-Krohn T, Truelson KA, Smith KP, et al. Screening for synergistic activity of antimicrobial combinations against carbapenem-resistant Enterobacteriaceae using inkjet printer-based technology. J Antimicrob Chemother 2017;72(10): 2775–81.
12. Smith KP, Kirby JE. How inkjet printing technology can defeat multidrug-resistant pathogens. Future Microbiol 2016;11:1375–7.
13. Smith KP, Kirby JE. Verification of an automated, digital dispensing platform for at-will broth microdilution-based antimicrobial susceptibility testing. J Clin Microbiol 2016;54(9):2288–93.
14. Brennan-Krohn T, Pironti A, Kirby JE. Synergistic activity of colistin-containing combinations against colistin-resistant enterobacteriaceae. Antimicrob Agents Chemother 2018;62(10) [pii:e00873-18].
15. Humphries RM, Hindler JA, Epson E, et al. carbapenem-resistant Enterobacteriaceae detection practices in California: what are we missing? Clin Infect Dis 2018;66(7):1061–7.
16. Regulation of laboratory developed tests (LDTs) (Policy Number 10-02). American Society for Clinical Pathology. 2016. Available at: https://www.ascp.org/content/docs/default-source/policy-statements/ascp-pdft-pp-regulation-of-ltds.pdf?sfvrsn=0. Accessed April 5, 2019.

17. Foodborne diseases active surveillance network (FoodNet). Atlanta, GA: US Centers for Disease Control and Prevention; 2018. Available at: https://www.cdc.gov/foodnet/index.html. Accessed April 5, 2019.

18. Surveillance and data systems. Atlanta, GA: US Centers for Disease Control and Prevention; 2018. Available at: https://www.cdc.gov/ncezid/dfwed/keyprograms/surveillance.html. Accessed April 5, 2019.

19. What is PulseNet? Association of public health laboratories. 2016. Available at: http://www.aphlblog.org/what-is-pulsenet/. Accessed April 5, 2019.

20. TBnet. 2019. Available at: http://www.tb-net.org/index.php/home. Accessed April 5, 2019.

21. Carrion M, Madoff LC. ProMED-mail: 22 years of digital surveillance of emerging infectious diseases. Int Health 2017;9(3):177–83.

22. Madoff LC. ProMED-mail: an early warning system for emerging diseases. Clin Infect Dis 2004;39(2):227–32.

23. Influenza: FluNet. Geneva (Switzerland): World Health Organization; 2019. Available at: https://www.who.int/influenza/gisrs_laboratory/flunet/en/. Accessed April 5, 2019.

24. Fuhrmeister AS, Jones RN. The importance of antimicrobial resistance monitoring Worldwide and the Origins of SENTRY antimicrobial surveillance program. Open Forum Infect Dis 2019;6(Suppl 1):S1–4.

25. ATLAS: Antimicrobial testing Leadership and surveillance. Available at: https://atlas-surveillance.com/. Accessed April 25, 2019.

26. Ben-David D, Masarwa S, Fallach N, et al. Success of a national intervention in controlling carbapenem-resistant Enterobacteriaceae in Israel's long-term care facilities. Clin Infect Dis 2019;68(6):964–71.

Pictorial Illustration

What Is the Future of Clinical Microbiology?

Alexander J. McAdam, MD, PhD

KEYWORDS

- Clinical microbiology • Polymerase chain reaction
- Matrix-assisted laser desorption ionization time of flight mass spectrometry
- Antimicrobial synergy

KEY POINTS

- There has been tremendous progress in clinical microbiology in the past 10 years.
- New technology has an important role in diagnosis of infectious diseases; however, it can be difficult to assess the utility of a new method when it is initially described.
- Potential benefits to new technologies include reduced turnaround time, improved sensitivity or specificity, and reduced cost.

In this comic, Strep and Staph consider the future of clinical microbiology. CRISPR-Cas, clustered regularly interspaced short palindromic repeats and CRISPR-associated protein; MALDI-TOF, matrix-assisted laser desorption ionization time-of-flight mass spectrometry; PCR, polymerase chain reaction; thio, thioglycollate.

Disclosure: Dr A.J. McAdam is a paid member of the Scientific Advisory Board for BacterioScan, Incorporated.
Department of Laboratory Medicine, Infectious Diseases Diagnostic Laboratory, Boston Children's Hospital, Harvard Medical School, 300 Longwood Avenue, Farley 7, Boston, MA 02115, USA
E-mail address: Alexander.McAdam@childrens.harvard.edu

Strep and Staph Consider the Future

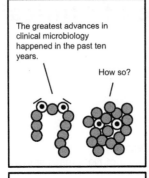

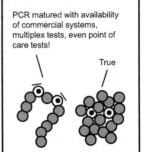

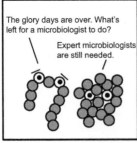

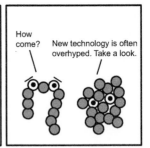

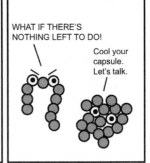

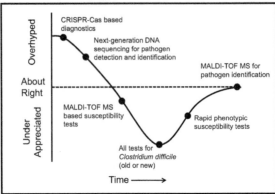

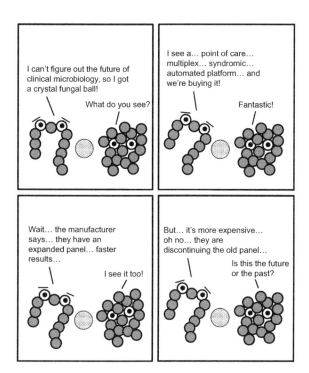

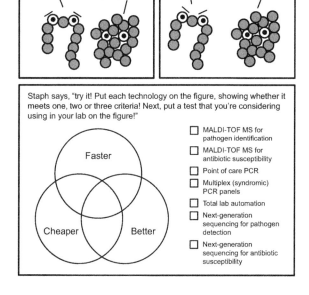

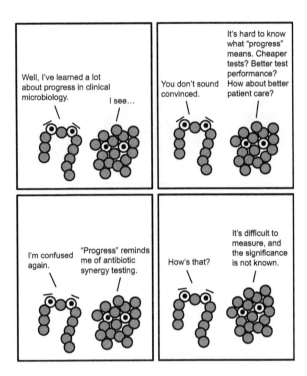

Moving?

Make sure your subscription moves with you!

To notify us of your new address, find your **Clinics Account Number** (located on your mailing label above your name), and contact customer service at:

Email: journalscustomerservice-usa@elsevier.com

800-654-2452 (subscribers in the U.S. & Canada)
314-447-8871 (subscribers outside of the U.S. & Canada)

Fax number: 314-447-8029

Elsevier Health Sciences Division
Subscription Customer Service
3251 Riverport Lane
Maryland Heights, MO 63043

*To ensure uninterrupted delivery of your subscription, please notify us at least 4 weeks in advance of move.

by CPI Group (UK) Ltd, Croydon, CR0 4YY

13/10/2024

01773503-0003